# Breastfeeding W

## A Breastfeeding Guide for Mothers through Adoption, Surrogacy, and Other Special Circumstances

Alyssa Schnell, MS, IBCLC

The companion website for this book can be found at: www.BreastfeedingWithoutBirthing.com.

Praeclarus Press, LLC

Praeclarus Press, LLC
2504 Sweetgum Lane
Amarillo, Texas 79124 USA
806-367-9950
www.PraeclarusPress.com

**DISCLAIMER**

The information contained in this publication is advisory only and is not intended to replace sound clinical judgment or individualized patient care. The author disclaims all warranties, whether expressed or implied, including any warranty as the quality, accuracy, safety, or suitability of this information for any particular purpose.

ISBN: 978-1-939807-00-7

ISBN (e-book): 978-1-939807-01-4

Cover Design and Illustration: Ken Tackett

Cover Author Photo: Mia Ulmer

Developmental Editing: Kathleen Kendall-Tackett

Copy Editing: Diana Cassar-Uhl

Layout & Design: Todd Rollison

Operations: Scott Sherwood

To Rosa, child of my heart

# Table of Contents

# SECTION III
# MAKING MILK—NOURISHING FROM THE BREAST

# FOREWORD

What a wonderful book for breastfeeding mothers! As an International Board Certified Lactation Consultant, I've worked with many mothers who wanted to breastfeed without birthing for many different reasons. My heart has always warmed to know that one more baby will have a breastfeeding experience with his mother. Your path to breastfeeding may not have been traditional, but all that matters to your baby is that you'll be offering the closeness, security, and reassurance of breastfeeding at a time when it matters most.

Were you surprised to learn that breastfeeding without birthing is possible? It's not quite mainstream yet, so the first time people hear about it, they can have very mixed reactions. Maybe you weren't too sure yourself at first, or maybe you have family members or friends who think it sounds strange.

Many years ago, I remember meeting the representative at my local bank. She knew that I had written a book for breastfeeding mothers, so she shyly mentioned that she was planning on adopting a baby and was thinking about, um, breastfeeding. Did I know of any ways to make it possible? I told her how wonderful it was that she was considering it, and I shared what I knew at the time, including the resources of La Leche League. But what we knew back then was nothing compared to the wonderful depth of resources that Alyssa offers in the book you're holding now. We didn't know very much about ways to start milk production without birth. We didn't know very much about ways to supplement at the breast. And we really didn't have much experience from people who had done it. Thankfully, the breastfeeding world has come a long way since then, and Alyssa has pulled together all the best information from many corners into one very readable and accessible resource.

*Breastfeeding Without Birthing* will be your companion as you work through the steps toward your breastfeeding relationship. And as an unofficial companion to this book, there are also communities of breastfeeding-without-birthing mothers to support each other, both online and in person. And there's a much wider community of breastfeeding supporters throughout the world who absolutely get why you want to do it and will be there for you as you go through your journey. So even if you don't have support at home, you're now automatically a member of the breastfeeding community, with all the honors, rights, and privileges (support! commiseration! tips and tricks!) pertaining thereto. Congratulations!

The one message I'd like to share with you is that it's important to focus on the positive whenever possible. In breastfeeding without birthing, as with many kinds of breastfeeding challenges, the road isn't always smooth, so having a "breast is half full" perspective can make all the difference in how you feel about your day-to-day experience. Nursing is about so much more than feeding. Focusing on the positive aspects of what you *can* give to your baby through breastfeeding is much more helpful to keeping things going long-term than worrying about the parts that aren't going as well you might wish they could.

With that said, I'll wish you a warm welcome to motherhood and to breastfeeding! You've joined a wonderful community of breastfeeding mothers around the world who are nursing their babies. If you ever feel alone, just think of how many moms are nursing their babies at this very minute. It may not always be easy, but what your baby needs most is simply being in your arms, surrounded by your never-ending love.

Diana West, BA, IBCLC
Author of *Defining Your Own Success:*
*Breastfeeding after Breast Reduction Surgery*,
Co-author of *The Breastfeeding Mother's*
*Guide to Making More Milk*,
and *The Womanly Art of Breastfeeding, 8th edition*

# ACKNOWLEDGEMENTS

Without you, Rosa, this book would never have been. Without you, Jonah and Cole, I would not have fallen so in love with breast-feeding that I knew breastfeeding would be a part of my parenting when I adopted. And my dear husband, Brad, who has loved me and our children, and who has been the ideal breastfeeding partner all the way. Thanks to all of you for your patience and support throughout the writing of this book.

Many, many thanks to all of my amazing colleagues who have been so generous in their support with this book. I would especially like to thank Diana Cassar-Uhl, Catherine Watson Genna, Karleen Gribble, Dee Kassing, Kathleen Kendall-Tackett, Amber McCann, Jack Newman, Barbara Wilson-Clay, and Diana West. Thank you to the product vendors who loaned their expertise (as well as their support): Silencia Cox at Motherlove Herbals and Joan Ortiz of Limerick, Inc. Thanks to Danielle Pennel from Adoptive Families Circle for being my adoption expert. Thank you to La Leche League, to my Leaders and co-Leaders over these last 16 years. A special thanks to colleague and co-Leader Laurie Shornick for all your help with the research for this book.

To all of the adoptive, intended, and other special mothers who have shared their breastfeeding journey with me ... it has been a privilege. Your stories have touched and inspired me. This book is both for you and thanks to you.

# INTRODUCTION

Congratulations! By simply picking up this book, you have taken the first step toward breastfeeding without first being pregnant or giving birth. In developed countries today, this is not a well-worn path, but it is one that you and I will travel together. The research and experiences of others before you have paved the way, and this book will put all of that together for you in a package that is clear, direct, specific, and supportive.

Every mother and baby deserves the chance to breastfeed. Even if that baby did not grow in that mother's uterus. Even if that baby is not a newborn. Even if that mother is not fertile. We are incredible, adaptive beings. Breastfeeding without birthing is one amazing example.

## Breastfeeding Without Birthing Defined

Breastfeeding without birthing is a term that emerged one evening as I was talking to my friend, Mia, at a party. I told her that I was looking for a term that was more inclusive than adoptive breastfeeding or adoptive nursing, since other mothers besides adoptive mothers breastfeed without giving birth. I explained further that the term induced lactation didn't quite work either, because it sounded so clinical to me. Even more importantly, breastfeeding is so much more than lactation: breastfeeding is also about the close connection that happens between mother and baby at the breast. "Sounds like you are talking about breastfeeding without birth," said Mia. Exactly.

## Breastfeeding-Without-Birthing Mothers

This book is for a variety of special mothers who did not birth their baby and who want to breastfeed:

- **Adoptive Mother.** The adoptive mother addressed in this book is a mother who has adopted a newborn, an older baby, or a toddler whom she wishes to breastfeed.

- **Intended Mother.** An intended mother is a mother whose baby is born via surrogacy. An intended mother will take a very similar breastfeeding route as an adoptive mother, but her circumstances are simpler and more certain. An intended mother has more certainty that plans will follow through, more certainty of timing, and will always begin with a newborn.

While this book primarily focuses on the circumstances of adoptive and intended mothers, several other special groups of mothers may also benefit. These include foster mothers and non-gestational lesbian mothers. They also include relactating or exclusively pumping mothers who have birthed, but they haven't *just* birthed. These mothers by birth are not currently breastfeeding, but they may wish to. Each of these special mothers will find much-needed information here, but may have some unique circumstances that reach beyond the scope of this book.

- **Foster Mother.** A foster mother is intended to serve the temporary role as mother until permanent placement can be made for the baby. In some cases, the permanent placement will be with the foster mother. Either way, it is not generally accepted or recommended for a foster mother to breastfeed. However, in certain circumstances, breastfeeding these special babies may be advisable. (See sidebar, When a Foster Mother May Choose to Breastfeed, for more information.)

- **Non-Gestational Lesbian Mother.** The baby of lesbian parents may be breastfed by her gestational mother as well as her non-gestational mother in a breastfeeding scenario sometimes called "co-breastfeeding" or "co-nursing." The non-gestational mother may choose to induce lactation, to supplement with her partner's expressed milk using a feeding tube at the breast, or to suckle her baby for comfort while her partner breastfeeds for nourishment.

- **Relactating Mother.** The relactating mother is a mother who birthed her baby and who is not currently making milk, but would like to. A relactating mother may have terminated breastfeeding because she was ill or required a medication, such as chemotherapy, that is incompatible with breastfeeding[1]; she may have originally decided against breastfeeding, but her baby has failed to thrive on infant formula; she may have stopped breastfeeding due to difficulties, but then regretted her decision; or any number of individual reasons.

- **Exclusively Pumping Mother.** The exclusively pumping mother is producing milk for her baby. She expresses her milk with a breast pump throughout the day, and then bottle-feeds her baby her expressed milk. For some mothers, this arrangement works. Other mothers, however, may wish to feed their babies directly from their breasts. Feeding at the

[1] It is very rare for a woman to need to stop breastfeeding because she must take a medication. Most medications are compatible with breastfeeding. Check with your lactation consultant before taking any medication while breastfeeding.

breast is much more convenient than pumping and bottle-feeding, and it can help a mother to feel closer to her baby. Just as adoptive and foster mothers may wish to teach an older baby to latch at the breast, an exclusively pumping mother can use the same approaches and tools.

## When a Foster Mother May Choose To Breastfeed

Although valid objections to breastfeeding a foster child exist, breastfeeding may still be the best choice for these special babies in certain circumstances.

During foster care, the baby is usually under the legal guardianship of the state. As such, if a foster mother were to breastfeed and, if any diseases were passed to the baby via the foster mother's milk, the foster mother or fostering agency could be held liable. A foster mother—just like any mother—should not breastfeed in certain circumstances in which her milk would be unsafe for the baby[2]. Yet, when no contraindications to breastfeeding exist, breastfeeding is considerably healthier for the baby than infant formula--especially when we consider that a high proportion of foster babies are medically fragile due to drug exposure in utero (Gribble, 2005).

Because many babies who enter the foster system are ill, there is some risk that disease may be passed from the baby

[2] Contraindications for breastfeeding are a baby with galactosemia or a mother with any of the following conditions: human immunodeficiency virus (HIV); human t-cell lymphotrophic virus (HTLV) type 1 or type 2; or untreated, active tuberculosis. Mothers taking antiretroviral medications, using an illicit drug, or undergoing chemotherapy or radiation therapy also should not breastfeed (CDC, 2009).

to the foster mother. Detailed medical history of the baby, birthmother, and foster mother can be collected to determine whether any such risk exists in a particular case (Gribble, 2005).

Finally, there is some concern that breastfeeding would cause the baby to become so attached to her foster mother that an eventual separation would be emotionally devastating, especially for a child who has already experienced separation and loss of her birthmother. On the contrary, research has shown that a child is better able to form an attachment to a new caregiver when she has already experienced a secure attachment with a prior caregiver than when she has experienced no attachment with a prior caregiver (Gribble, 2005).

Although valid objections exist, breastfeeding may still be the best choice. Karleen Gribble, Ph.D. (2005) has identified some specific circumstances in which a foster mother may choose to breastfeed.

1. The child is likely to be in long-term care with the family (six to 12 months). In such cases, breastfeeding would not disrupt the child's feeding routine (as might be the case in which a child quickly returns to the care of the birth family), but may greatly benefit the child.

2. The child was breastfed prior to placement in foster care, and continuing breastfeeding may assist the child in making the transition to foster care.

3. The biological mother expresses the desire that her child be breastfed. Some biological mothers, as part of the process of working toward regaining custody of their child,

may even maintain their milk supply with the intention of breastfeeding their child upon reunion. Maintaining the breastfeeding relationship with the foster mother can help facilitate a return to breastfeeding with the biological mother.

If you are a foster mother whose situation falls into one of these categories, it is recommended that you check with your local legal authorities before proceeding with breastfeeding.

### Maria's Story

*Maria was a foster mother to three-month-old Jada. Although Maria was an experienced breastfeeding mother, and had a strong desire to breastfeed Jada, it was against the regulations of the fostering agency. Maria respected these wishes. Jada was a very fussy baby who cried almost constantly. Maria tried everything that she knew to calm and comfort poor Jada. Then, one day as Maria was just coming from the shower, she rushed to pick up the crying Jada. Skin-to-skin against Maria's bare chest, Jada spontaneously started breastfeeding. For the first time since Jada had been living with Maria, Jada was calm and content. After that day, Maria found that Jada was a happy, content baby … as long as she was able to breastfeed.*

### Defining Breastfeeding

Although it may seem obvious, the breastfeeding community has struggled with a conclusive definition for "breastfeeding" for many years (Labbok, 2000). In this book, breastfeeding is defined as nourishing a baby with her mother's milk and/or nurturing a baby at her mother's breast. It is a deliberately broad definition. It includes the mother who:

- Provides 100% of her baby's food by suckling from her breast,
- Provides some of her baby's food by suckling from her breast, and offers the remainder as supplements of expressed milk or formula in a bottle or other feeding device,
- Produces little-to-no milk and feeds her baby using a device to deliver expressed milk or formula through a feeding tube attached to her breast (at-breast supplementer),
- Produces an abundant amount of milk that she pumps from her breasts and gives her baby in a bottle, or
- Comforts her little one at the breast without providing milk.

The combinations are endless. Every mother, baby, and situation is unique.

## Is Breastfeeding Without Birthing a New Idea?

Breastfeeding without birthing has happened since the beginning of time. Before the invention of infant formula or electric breast pumps, another woman, called a wet nurse, would breastfeed a baby when her mother was either unable to or was financially able to choose not to. In the 1600s and 1700s in North America, England, and some European countries, wealthy mothers would hire wet nurses to breastfeed their babies so that they would be free to attend to their social obligations (Riordan, 2005). Furthermore, when young mothers returned to work, it was not uncommon for the baby's grandmother to nurse the baby during the mother's absence. Breastfeeding without birthing is not a new idea, but it is uncommon in developed cultures today. This book is designed to make your breastfeeding experience a success even if the path has not been well traveled for quite a while.

## Keys to Success

Jelliffe and Jelliffe (1972), in their landmark letter in the journal *Pediatrics*, identified four keys to successful breastfeeding without giving birth: **knowledge, confidence, suckling, and stimulation of hormones**. *Breastfeeding Without Birthing* arms you with each of these tools.

### Chapter 1: How Important Is It?

We start out our breastfeeding adventure with the decision that breastfeeding is indeed a worthwhile endeavor. The first chapter of the book offers us the **knowledge** of how important breastfeeding is for our precious little one and for ourselves. The rest of the book offers the **knowledge** of how to make it happen. For mothers looking for even more **knowledge** beyond the scope of this book, my companion site: *www.BreastfeedingWithoutBirthing.com*, offers a list of additional resources.

### Section I: Creating Your Support Network

Jelliffe and Jelliffe (1972) suggest that the key to confidence is social support. Section I is devoted to developing your support networks, both personal and professional. Throughout the rest of the book, I have included numerous mothers' stories of breastfeeding without birthing, including plenty of my own. Breastfeeding without birthing is a bold journey, but you will not be traveling it alone.

## Allison's Story

I found this inspiring story in Barbara Behrmann's *The Breastfeeding Café* by a mother who adopted a baby with Down syndrome, who was also diagnosed as failing to thrive. Adoptive mother, Allison, shares her story.

> *I tried to nurse her and she latched on and sucked beautifully. I couldn't believe it! The feeling of looking down at this child, and seeing my white breast and her deep brown skin, with dark eyes looking up at me, was beyond description. But I didn't think she could be doing it right, so I continued to give her formula. Gradually, though, she drank less and less of it. After I'd been nursing her for about a week and a half, I started to panic. She was on this super-high-fat, high calorie formula, but now she was only drinking about an ounce a day. I took her to the doctor and found that she had gained about a pound. This was unbelievable! When we got her at ten weeks, she'd only weighed about an ounce more than when she was born. (Behrmann, 2005, pp. 99-100).*

## Section II: Latching – Nurturing at the Breast

**Suckling** your baby at the breast, more recently known as *latching* or simply *breastfeeding*, is the focus of Section II. We will discuss parenting practices that support your baby's ability to latch. For older babies, or any baby having difficulty learning to latch onto the breast, these chapters will help you through.

## Section III: Making Milk – Nourishing at the Breast

Breastfeeding is driven by hormones. Section III provides you with avenues for **stimulating the hormones** of lactation in order to develop breasts in preparation for lactation, and then to make and release milk from your breasts. We will discuss physical techniques, primarily breastfeeding (yes, **suckling** is emphasized here, too), and using a breast pump. We will also discuss pharmaceutical and herbal medications, as well as foods, to increase the effectiveness of the physical techniques.

# This Book's for You!

When my husband Brad and I decided to adopt, I immediately began researching how I could breastfeed this special baby. I had breastfed my two children by birth, and I knew that breastfeeding was such an important part of how I mother a baby. I was very lucky, because I had experience breastfeeding my other two children and because, as an accredited La Leche League leader, I had access to plenty of breastfeeding support, information, and resources. I thought about how most prospective adoptive and intended mothers did not have the head start on breastfeeding that I was privileged to have.

In the process of researching adoptive breastfeeding, I found a lovely–yet unlikely--book called *Defining Your Own Success: Breast-feeding After Breast Reduction Surgery*, written by Diana West, IBCLC. While it is a book for women who have had breast-reduction surgery, many of the issues facing these mothers overlapped with those faced by adoptive, intended, and other special mothers: maximizing milk production and the likely need to supplement breastfeeding. Not only was this book loaded with helpful information, Diana West shared it with a tone of compassion, honesty, gentleness, and warmth. I loved this book for these reasons, yet I couldn't help but think, "Where is *my* book?" Where was the informative and warm book for mothers like me? And *you*? Inspired by *Defining Your Own Success*, this book is for *us*.

# Chapter 1

# HOW IMPORTANT
# IS IT FOR YOU TO BREASTFEED?

Breastfeeding is important for mothers, and it is important for babies. With the exception of some uncommon maternal and infant medical conditions, all mothers *can* breastfeed their babies (ACOG, 2007; WHO, 2003). That includes mothers like us!

Breastfeeding promotes bonding between the mother and baby, provides essential infant nutrition, is required for the development of the baby's immune system, protects the health of the mother, and supports normal infant development. While each of these benefits of breastfeeding is so valuable for every mother/baby dyad, they are especially important for breastfeeding-without-birthing mothers and their babies.

## Breastfeeding Fosters Attachment
## Between Mother and Baby

No one who has ever seen a nursing child at his mother's breasts can doubt that, to a little person, breastfeeding is sheer delight. Skin to skin, with his mother's delicious smell enveloping his senses, a breastfed baby is frequently overcome with happiness as he nurses. He will pat or caress his mother's breast as he sucks, and older babies like to glance up at their mother's face and give a milky smile. These are the moments nursing mothers really treasure (Granju & Kennedy, 1999, p. 128).

Attachment is important for all children. For babies in traditional families, that attachment begins in utero and carries through after the child is born (Gribble, 2006). For babies who come to their parents via adoption, surrogacy, or foster care, the initial attachment that began with the gestational mother has been disrupted. The disruption may be brief, though still significant, as a baby is placed at birth into his adoptive or intended mother's arms. The disruption may be extensive, as when a

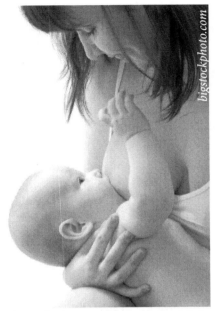

A breastfeeding mother and baby delight in each other's company. Essentially, breastfeeding is a relationship.

child is placed for several months--or even years--in an institutionalized setting with minimum human contact; when the child's parents are addicted to drugs or alcohol; when the parents suffer from depression or mental illness; or when the child experiences physical abuse, sexual abuse, or domestic violence (Clark et al., 2009). The degree of disruption your baby experienced may be somewhere in between.

Breastfeeding helps to heal your baby's break in attachment from his birth or surrogate mother, and helps your baby attach to you, because in essence, breastfeeding is a relationship. It fosters trust and connection between mother and baby in multiple ways.

- Breastfeeding means baby is frequently in close physical contact with his mother, one of the fundamental components of creating attachment.

- Because breasts don't contain measurements of how much milk is removed, mothers must be in tune to their babies' cues to determine when and for how long to feed them.

- Hormones released in both the mother and the baby during breastfeeding help create feelings of calm and connection between them (Moberg, 2003).

*The Womanly Art of Breastfeeding*, La Leche League's classic breast-feeding book, suggests that:

> … if you talk to most experienced breastfeeding mothers, they're more likely to focus on the way that breastfeeding helps you and your baby feel connected and attached to each other, weaving an emotional cord to replace the umbilical cord (Wiessinger et al., 2010, p. 10).

This observation is especially poignant to those of us who never were connected with our babies via the umbilical cord! One adoptive mother who breastfed her second adopted child, but not her first, described breastfeeding as "one of the best experiences of my life" and "worth every minute of frustration I experienced." She felt that she had established a special bond with her breastfed baby that she had not experienced with her first baby (Cheales-Siebenaler, 1999).

**My Story: Attachment begins in Utero**

*When my daughter Rosa was born, I had the opportunity to attend her birth and room with her and her birthmother during the hospital stay. During those couple of days, there were many visitors, most of whom were family and friends of her birthmother and knew this would likely be their only opportunity to meet Rosa. As these visitors held Rosa tenderly, admired her lovingly, and cooed at her, I observed Rosa's body language. She was stiff. Reserved. Rosa's birthmother chose to hold her only a few times during the hospital stay, because she knew that holding Rosa would make it more difficult to let her go. When Rosa's birthmother did hold her, she kept her distance emotionally, holding Rosa rigidly and coolly in her arms with little or no eye contact and without speaking directly to her. Yet, Rosa looked so much more comfortable with her birthmother than with anyone else who held her. "At home" was the best way I could describe the way she looked in her birthmother's arms.*

## Human Milk is the Normal Food for a Baby

Over 200 components of human milk have been identified and more are being recognized all the time. No other food contains all of the nutrients that a baby needs. No other food is designed just for human babies. Infant formula is available for our babies if human milk is not (WHO, 2003).

## Breastfeeding Protects Baby Against Illness

Newly adopted and foster babies are more likely to get sick. Adoption and breastfeeding expert, Dr. Karleen Gribble (2006), identifies numerous reasons why adoptive, intended, and foster mothers should consider breastfeeding to protect the health of their vulnerable babies:

- Adoption, foster care, and even surrogacy disrupt attachment, and disruption in attachment reduces resistance to disease (Maunder & Hunter, 2001).
- All newly adopted children are under considerable stress. Children under stress are more susceptible to illness (Drummund & Hewson-Bower, 1997; Wilson et al., 2003).
- Children adopted from another country are bombarded with a new set of viruses that they have not previously been exposed to (Schneider, 1986).
- Children in foster care have a higher-than-typical incidence of health issues (Halfon et al., 1995).
- A history of early trauma, such as abuse or neglect, can impact immune system function (Schleifer et al., 1986).

These early stresses on the immune system can impact your baby's current health, as well as your child's immune capacity over his lifetime (Schleifer et al., 1986).

A breastfeeding mother can provide the immunological protection that her baby needs, even if she doesn't produce a full milk supply. No matter how much milk a mother produces, a full set of antibodies is concentrated in the milk. Mother's milk contains antibodies to the viruses that the mother has been exposed to. When her baby has arrived from another country, the local antibodies contained in mother's milk are particularly important. Mother's milk can also contain antibodies to the viruses her baby is fighting: the baby will expose his mother to any virus he is carrying and then her body will respond by producing antibodies secreted in her milk.

# Breastfeeding Protects Mother's Health

Breastfeeding protects a mother's physical and emotional health. Non-gestational mothers may be at a higher risk for reproductive cancers due to lack of pregnancies. Breastfeeding provides protection against breast, ovarian, and uterine cancers (Collaborative Group on Hormonal Factors in Breast Cancer, 2002; Ip et al., 2007) Breastfeeding decreases mother's risk of cardiovascular diseases later in life, such as heart disease, high blood pressure, and stroke. It also protects mother's emotional health by releasing hormones into her system that reduce stress, improve relationships, and make her feel more nurturing. Postpartum depression can also happen to adoptive mothers, and breastfeeding can help (United States Department of Health and Human Services [HHS], 2013).

# Breastfeeding Supports Normal Infant Development

Babies who are adopted or are in foster care are at risk for developmental delays. Although not always the case, these babies were more likely to have suffered harm in utero due to lack of prenatal medical care; poor nutrition; and exposure to nicotine, alcohol, or recreational drugs. A baby can even be developmentally affected by the stress of his birthmother's unwanted pregnancy (Palmer, 2011). When older babies are adopted, they tend to be even more developmentally behind their peers (Gribble, 2004).

Breastfeeding aids normal development in a variety of ways. Suckling at the breast teaches babies how to properly use their tongues for swallowing and speaking, and promotes normal development of the bones of the palate and jaw (Palmer, 2011). The position of the baby during breastfeeding, and the fact that babies naturally feed facing in both directions, helps develop vision and eye-hand coordination. Components of human milk aid in brain development, resulting in lower IQ scores for children who were not breastfed (Jedrychowski et al., 2012).

## Breastfeeding Helps Heal the Heartache of Infertility

Breastfeeding can help mothers heal from the heartache of infertility. Many women become adoptive or intended mothers because they were unable to conceive or carry a baby. These mothers have experienced a great loss: the loss of a dream to bear a child. When her baby suckles at her breast and grows on her milk, the breastfeeding-without-birthing mother experiences a biological connection with her baby.

> While it is certainly true that mothers can love and feel close to their babies no matter how they feed them, the attachment between a breastfeeding mother and her nursling is more than just a feeling. In fact, this connection is tangible and biological, and is similar in many respects to the connection between a pregnant mother and the baby she is carrying. Anthropologists have determined that human infants—compared with other mammals—are exceptionally helpless and "unfinished" when they emerge from the womb. They still need the biological connection of breastfeeding for optimal development. Birth itself is not the end product of a new mother's reproductive cycle. For

both mother and baby, there is one last step to human gestation: breastfeeding (Granju & Kennedy, 1999, p. 124).

In the words of one mother,

> Breastfeeding was so worth it! I not only felt like most of my "broken" pieces weren't so important anymore--something maternal worked just like for other women--but being able to nurse in the presence of gestational moms leveled the playing field. It was like I was finally like other "normal" mothers (Davenport, 2012).

## Breastfeeding Aids the Baby's Transition

When an infant grieves the loss of his gestational mother or other caregivers, he responds somatically: either his digestion or his sleep may be negatively impacted (Melina, 1998). When an older child is having digestive difficulties, parents will offer them foods that are more easily digestible. The same logic is true for babies. Infant formula causes difficulties with digestion that human milk isn't likely to cause. Human milk is the perfect food for sensitive little tummies.

Breastfeeding is also an excellent remedy for sleep problems. Components in human milk are relaxants and will help baby fall asleep. The act of breastfeeding reduces the infant's stress levels, also helping him sleep better.

## What is Important to You?

While I have listed reasons why breastfeeding without birthing can be so important, some reasons will surely feel more important to you than others. I encourage you to think about your personal reasons for wanting to breastfeed your baby. You may even want to rank the reasons in order of importance to you so that you can base your breastfeeding plan on these priorities. (You may find that they change over time–and that's okay!) Keep your list of reasons nearby to offer you encouragement along the journey.

## Section I

# Creating Your Support Network

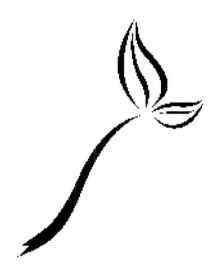

# Chapter 2
# A COMMUNITY OF SUPPORT

Establishing a support network is the first and arguably the most important step for any mother planning to breastfeed. For mothers who are breastfeeding under special circumstances, the support network becomes even more crucial. You will need some specialized support in addition to the general support that all breastfeeding mothers need. Some of those who can provide support are people you already know and who care about you. Some are people you can seek out, and I'll tell you how.

## Support of Family and Friends

### Partner

Your partner, if you have one, may be the most important source of breastfeeding and mothering support (HHS, 2011). That goes for all mothers, not just breastfeeding-without-birthing mothers. In fact, partners have an entire chapter written just for them devoted to how they can support you. I encourage you to ask your partner to read Chapter 3, Especially For Partners: You Make a Difference.

### Other Family Members and Friends

When any mother brings a new baby home, the support of family and friends is invaluable. They can help with meals, housework, and the care of older children. In cases in which you will need to travel to meet your child, support back home can be even more essential.

# Mother-to-Mother Support

Being with other breastfeeding mothers is how we are meant to learn to breastfeed.

### Breastfeeding Friends and Family Members

Let's start with some people you already know: mothers in your life who have successfully breastfed or, even better, who are currently breastfeeding their babies. These people include your friends and family members, such as your sister, mother, sister-in-law, mother-in-law, etc. According to the U.S. Surgeon General, "women with friends who have breastfed successfully are more likely to choose to breastfeed" (HHS, 2011, p. 12). Your friends are likely to want to share their stories with you and offer you valuable encouragement and support in your breastfeeding plans. On the contrary, "negative attitudes of family and friends can pose a barrier to breastfeeding" (HHS, 2011, p. 12). You know who will be able to support you well.

### Breastfeeding Mothers' Groups

In Western countries, many mothers find that they don't have rich resources of breastfeeding support within their group of family and friends. Our culture does not yet have enough women who are successfully breastfeeding. This is where breastfeeding mothers' groups can be extremely helpful—even essential—to breastfeeding success.

Research on adoptive breastfeeding has shown that mothers in developing countries are much more likely to produce sufficient quantities of milk than mothers in Western countries (Gribble,

2004). Instead of resigning to these findings, you can emulate some of the parenting styles in developing countries that support success-ful induced lactation. These parenting styles can be absorbed within the breastfeeding-supportive culture of breastfeeding mothers' groups (Thorley, 2004).

The original breastfeeding mothers' group is La Leche League International (LLLI). La Leche League has breastfeeding mothers' groups all over the world, and continues to be a leading resource for mother-to-mother support, information, and encouragement for breastfeeding. You may find that your community has other resources for mother-to-mother support as well, such as Nursing Mothers Council, Breastfeeding USA, hospital-based breastfeeding groups, retail-based breastfeeding groups, WIC, or individual groups led by board certified lactation consultants.

## Allison's Story: LLLove

*When Allison made the decision to breastfeed her adopted baby, she was already a longtime member of La Leche League. La Leche League had supported Allison through breastfeeding challenges with her two biological babies. It was natural for her to share her breastfeeding plans with her La Leche League group and, as they always had, her LLL friends overflowed with support and encouragement. They believed she could do this when Allison wasn't so sure herself.*

*As Allison walked into one LLL meeting while she was in the process of inducing lactation before her baby arrived, her LLL leader Tammy's eyes widened. Motioning toward Allison's swelling chest, Tammy chuckled, "I can see that inducing lactation is working!" Allison hadn't noticed that her breasts had grown in preparation for lactation, but her LLL leader had.*

As important as breastfeeding support is, I'd like to add a word of caution. Before stepping into a La Leche League meeting, or a meeting of another breastfeeding mothers' group, consider how you may feel seeing pregnant women, hearing birth stories, or simply seeing women who easily produce plenty of milk. When they learn you are breastfeeding without birthing, you are likely to find a lot of encouragement. You may still find it emotionally difficult to see other mothers sharing experiences that you wished that you could have. If so, you may be able to find a La Leche League leader or other group leader who is willing to meet with you one-on-one to offer you support.

**Breastfeeding-Without-Birthing Mothers**

Sometimes, mothers are more comfortable and find it more helpful to be with other mothers experiencing special breastfeeding circumstances like their own. In rare cases, communities may have breastfeeding groups for breastfeeding-without-birthing mothers. If not, you may be able to create your own little group by connecting with just one or two local adoptive or intended mothers who are currently or planning to breastfeed. You may be able to find these women via the breastfeeding route (check with your local breastfeeding experts, such as board certified lactation consultants or La Leche League leaders), or the adoption/surrogacy route (check with your local adoption/surrogacy professionals).

You can also find an online group of breastfeeding-without-birthing mothers. Be careful, however, when gleaning breastfeeding information from online groups. Most are not monitored by a trained breastfeeding expert, such as a board certified lactation consultant or a La Leche League leader. In searching through these online groups, I have frequently come across incorrect breastfeeding information provided by a non-professional. On the other hand, the mothers on these online groups can be so incredibly supportive of one another—they understand because they have been there too! See the Links page on my website to connect to an online group of breastfeeding-without-birthing mothers.

## When Others are Critical

When you let others know that you will be, or already are, breastfeeding a baby you haven't birthed, most people will be impressed and quite amazed. You will find most people are very supportive because they know breastfeeding really makes a difference for babies. Some people, though, will be extremely uncomfortable with the idea. They may believe that it is unnatural, even sexually abusive, to suckle a baby who was not born to you. They may believe that the milk you produce is an "abnormal diet of your hormone-induced cocktail," and is therefore a dangerous food for your baby (Davenport, 2011). While scientific research, endorsements by medical and mental health professionals, as well as the experience of mothers who have breastfed a baby they didn't birth contradict these perceptions, they can still hurt. You are reading this book because you want to nourish and nurture your baby in the best way possible, and any indication to the contrary is painful. How can you handle concerns or even harsh criticism? The following page contains some things that may help.

- **Consider the Source.** When critical comments stem from true concern for your well-being or that of your baby, thank the person for caring and acknowledge his or her feelings. Breastfeeding without birthing is a new idea for most people and can take some getting used to. Sometimes critical comments are not well meaning. In that case, they are probably about the insecurities of the person saying them, and not really about you or your baby at all. Take a few deep breaths and let it go as best you can. Take care of yourself by turning to those people who are supportive.

- **Provide Information.** Scientific research overwhelmingly supports the emotional, mental, and physical health benefits to the baby of breastfeeding without birthing. Breastfeeding promotes attachment: it helps your baby to feel safe, secure, and connected to you—the opposite of abuse. This book recommends a gentle and respectful transition to breastfeeding, never forcing or coercing as in abuse. Furthermore, the milk of a mother who has induced lactation has all of the same wonderful nutritional and immunological components as that of a mother who has birthed (Kulski et al., 1981). It does not contain any artificial hormones (unless mother is taking them for a reason unrelated to inducing lactation). At no point in researching this book have I found any reported harm to a baby who drank the milk of his mother who induced lactation.

> • **Quote the Experts**. A doctor's opinion garners a lot of respect, so let your doctor make the case for you: "My pediatrician is thrilled that I'm breastfeeding my baby." The American Academy of Pediatrics statement of support (see below) may also be helpful.

## Support of the Gestational Family

### Birth Family

Adoption plans can be very emotionally difficult for the birth family. Throwing your breastfeeding plans into the mix can be an added hurdle for them. Most birth families will not be expecting to hear about your intention to breastfeed, and will need some time to adjust to the idea. Until the birth parents have signed the consent for adoption[1], the baby is still their child and it is imperative that you honor their wishes regarding the feeding of their baby, even if they are contrary to breastfeeding success. Even if the birth family expresses their support of your decision to breastfeed, consider how emotionally difficult it may be for your baby's birthmother to witness you sharing the intimate relationship of breastfeeding with this baby she has just birthed. Once the birth parents have released their parental rights and the baby is in your custody, of course, how you feed your baby is your choice.

---

[1] Each state determines when the birth parents can sign the consent for adoption. This timing varies considerably from state to state, although most states allow birthparents to consent at 48 hours, 72 hours, or sooner after the birth (HHS, 2010).

41

## Ruby's Story: Jump Start to Breastfeeding

*Soon after baby Michael was born, his prospective adoptive mother, Ruby, put him to the breast. Ruby knew that offering the breast soon after birth is the best way to initiate breastfeeding. While Michael latched onto Ruby's breast without difficulty, Michael's birthmother reported that seeing Michael at Ruby's breast was too emotionally difficult for her. Michael's mother decided to cancel her adoption plans. Later, Ruby was matched with another baby. Again she put the baby to her breast in the hospital soon after the birth, and again the birthmother canceled her adoption decision. When Ruby was matched a third time, she did not attempt to latch baby Nicholas until adoption papers were signed and they were home from the hospital.*

## Surrogate Mother

Although some intended mothers may choose to breastfeed their babies right from birth, others may request that the surrogate mother breastfeed the baby or express milk (by hand or with a breast pump) for the first few days following birth so that the baby receives the nutrient-rich and immunity-dense first milk, called colostrum. (Mothers who induce lactation do not generally produce significant amounts of colostrum, if any at all.) Some parents may also request that their surrogate pump milk for a specified period of time to provide for the baby once they return home. These are some considerations to communicate with your surrogate attorney about, and to negotiate when choosing a potential surrogate.

# Support of the Healthcare Team

Your healthcare team may be a diverse combination of those healthcare professionals caring for the birth or surrogate mother, for the baby, and for you. It is not realistic to expect any of these healthcare professionals besides your board certified lactation consultant to know much, if anything, about breastfeeding without birthing. It is likely that you will be the person educating them about it. What is important is that these healthcare professionals are receptive and supportive of your plans.

### Your Lactation Consultant

Professional breastfeeding support should come from an International Board Certified Lactation Consultant (IBCLC). According to the U.S. Surgeon General,

> International Board Certified Lactation Consultants are the only healthcare professionals certified in lactation care (2011, p. 27).

The time to schedule your first meeting with your lactation consultant is as soon as you are considering breastfeeding. A lactation consultant can answer any questions you might have, work with you to develop your breastfeeding-without-birthing plan, and provide guidance along the way. Not all lactation consultants have experience working with breastfeeding-without-birthing mothers: don't hesitate to ask if there is an expert in this area in your community.

IBCLCs can be found in the following settings:

- **Private Practice:** Most successful breastfeeding-without-birthing mothers attain help from an IBCLC in private practice. These helpers are likely to spend the time to work with you in detail and develop a personal relationship with you. Many of them have worked with breastfeeding-without-birthing mothers in the past.

- **Hospitals:** If you are with your baby when she is born in the hospital, you may be able to work with the IBCLCs on staff there. Some hospitals also offer outpatient lactation services. For those that do, they may only be available to mothers who gave birth in that hospital. If you are able to contact the hospital before your baby is born, you can determine what type of lactation support is available for you.
- **WIC:** WIC is the U.S. Federal Government's supplemental nutrition program for low-income pregnant, breastfeeding, and postpartum women, along with their infants and children up to age five. For mothers who qualify, WIC provides support for breastfeeding by offering lactation counseling, breast pumps, and other breastfeeding accessories for little to no cost.

If you will be traveling to meet your baby, look into finding an IBCLC wherever you will be staying, especially if you will be staying out of town for longer than your baby's hospital stay.

**Your Doctor**

Your doctor, either your primary care physician or your obstetrician/gynecologist, plays a vital role in your breastfeeding success.

- Your approach to breastfeeding without birthing may require your doctor to write a prescription or evaluate the safety of medications for you. Certainly, a supportive attitude from your doctor is helpful here.
- Breastfeeding affects, and is affected by, your health. Your

doctor can help you understand your health history, and your lactation consultant can help you understand how this history may influence your ability to produce milk. If you have experienced difficulties with fertility due to hormonal issues, these same issues may have an impact on lactation. (See Chapter 9, Making Milk: What to Expect.)

- Your doctor can also help you achieve a healthy hormonal balance to support optimum lactation outcomes. Traditional doctors may suggest medications, and complementary and alternative healthcare practitioners, such as chiropractors, homeopaths, naturopaths, acupuncturists, herbalists, or doctors of Chinese medicine may be able to offer natural routes to hormonal balance.

## Your Baby's Doctor

Your baby's doctor can support your breastfeeding success, or he can undermine it. Although pediatricians receive little-to-no education in breastfeeding while in medical school, many pediatricians have seen for themselves the importance of breastfeeding to a baby's health. When interviewing pediatricians, try to determine whether your pediatrician is breastfeeding-friendly by asking the following:

- What percentage of the patients in your practice are breastfeeding at six weeks, six months, and into toddlerhood? (Granju & Kennedy, 1999; Kuhn, 1999).
- Does the office have an International Board Certified Lactation Consultant (IBCLC) on staff or an IBCLC that they will refer patients to? (In my experience, some pediatrician offices say that they have a "lactation consultant" on staff, but they really have a nurse, not an IBCLC.)

45

- Does the office have promotional or "educational" materials provided by infant formula companies (Granju & Kennedy, 1999)? These types of materials undermine breastfeeding success.
- Did you/your wife/partner breastfeed?

## My Story: Rosa's First Doctor Visit

*When I first brought Rosa to see the family doctor at two weeks old, she was well above her birthweight. Upon seeing her chart, the doctor gently asked me in several different ways what else I was feeding her in addition to breastfeeding. I finally convinced him that Rosa was exclusively breastfed. He just sat there and stared at me for a minute or so, then abruptly stood up and dashed from the room. He returned a few minutes later with the nurse practitioner. "You've got to see this!" he exclaimed to her. From our quiet and reserved family doc of many years, this response was totally out of character. That was all the encouragement that I could ask for!*

The American Academy of Pediatrics (AAP) supports your decision to breastfeed. Their 2005 Policy Statement, *Breastfeeding and the Use of Human Milk*, states that pediatricians should:

> ... provide counsel to adoptive mothers who decide to breastfeed through induced lactation, a process requiring professional support and encouragement (AAP, 2005, p. 501).

The AAP's press release announcing the 2005 Policy Statement further states:

Pediatricians should counsel adoptive mothers on the benefits of induced lactation through hormonal therapy or mechanical stimulation (Davenport, 2009).

## The Hospital Medical Staff and Hospital Policies

If you will be attending your baby's birth or participating during the hospital stay, find out (ahead of time, if possible) what the hospital policies are regarding your rights to breastfeed. With adoption, breastfeeding during the hospital stay can be a bit complicated. Hospitals may only allow the baby to receive her birthmother's milk or infant formula until the birth parents have signed consent for adoption. Before the paperwork is signed, the birthmother can change her mind, and the hospital may be liable if another mother has breastfed the baby. The adoptive mother is not a patient, and therefore the hospital has no medical records for her. Even if allowed by the hospital, it may still not be sensitive or advisable to breastfeed until the birth parents have consented and the baby is in your custody.

With surrogacy, your pre-birth order may specify you as the legal parent which, in this case, gives you the right to determine how your baby will be fed from the start.

In any case, if breastfeeding will be initiated at birth in the delivery room, the delivering obstetrician and hospital pediatrician should be notified beforehand, if possible. A forewarning can help prevent them from making any objections to this out-of-the-ordinary situation. It may (or may not) also help for your baby's (future) doctor to write an order requesting your milk or, if possible, banked milk (from a nonprofit milk bank) be fed to the baby during the hospital stay.

It can help to inform the hospital staff regarding your plans to breastfeed, even if you will not be breastfeeding in the hospital. They may be able to support you in other ways: providing a place for you to pump, allowing you to use one of the hospital's breast pumps, providing refrigerator storage space for your expressed milk, helping you to feed your baby-to-be in a way that supports breastfeeding, and not offering a pacifier.

### My Story: The Breastfeeding Sneak

*The policy of the hospital where Rosa was born required the baby be fed her birthmother's milk or formula until the adoption paperwork was signed. Since her birthmother, understandably, did not choose to breastfeed Rosa, Rosa was fed formula during the hospital stay. All the while, I pumped and stored my milk every few hours. It was heartbreaking to feed my baby an inferior food knowing I had the good stuff "in stock!" One night in the hospital, when Rosa woke up hungry, and I prepared to feed her formula and then pump, I decided it was just ridiculous! I offered her my breast. Nervous as I was, and sitting in the dark so as not to disturb Rosa's birthmother and birthgrandmother, I could not get her to latch. Just as I gave up and pulled down my pajama top, the nurse walked in. How could I have potentially risked my adoption arrangement just to start breastfeeding one day early?*

## Support from Your Professional Team

Let your professional team know that you plan to breastfeed. This includes adoption and surrogacy professionals, social workers, and lawyers. These professionals may be able to foster communication with a birthmother, advocate for you with the hospital, or even connect you with sources of support. My adoption professional helped

A Community of Support

me connect with another adoptive mother who had successfully breastfed. In the case of surrogacy, breastfeeding plans can be part of the pre-birth order, especially if your plans involve the surrogate mother breastfeeding during the hospital stay or pumping her milk for your baby.

### Books and the Internet

> ... find real, live people ... You would never learn to swim or ride a bicycle by going to the Internet (Wiessinger, 2008).

Books and the Internet cannot replace the support of live people, but they do have an important place. Sometimes people provide contradictory information, which can make breastfeeding more difficult, rather than less (HHS, 2011). A well-researched book can set the record straight. Reading this book is a great start! Supplementing this book with an excellent general-purpose breastfeeding book will round out your breastfeeding resources by addressing the aspects of breastfeeding that are universal among breastfeeding mothers. Written and online resources can provide information in a clear and organized fashion, be research-based, and are available to you at 3:00 a.m. when you've got a breastfeeding issue that just can't wait! See my website Library pages for a listing of recommended general breastfeeding books, and my Links page to connect with online sources of breastfeeding information.

49

# Chapter 3

## ESPECIALLY FOR PARTNERS: YOU MAKE A DIFFERENCE

This chapter is devoted to you, the non-breastfeeding parenting partner. You may be the father, co-mother, or a close friend or family member who is sharing parenting responsibilities. By whatever name you are called, you can provide the most important breastfeeding support for your partner. It may seem that breastfeeding falls solely into the realm of the breastfeeding mother, but the partner is a vital component of the breastfeeding team. When couples approach breastfeeding as a team, the breastfeeding mother's job becomes much easier and more rewarding. When partners are educated about breastfeeding and play a supportive role, breastfeeding is more likely to happen and to happen for a longer period of time (HHS, 2011; Pisacane et al., 2005; Tohotoa et al., 2009). While this book predominantly addresses mothers because they play the primary role in breastfeeding, it is essential that we include you, the partner, and the immensely valuable role that you play in breastfeeding success.

**Offer Encouragement**

Tell her you believe in her. Tell her she is doing an amazing job. Tell her she can do it!

**When there is No Partner**

Many mothers have successful breastfeeding experiences without a partner. Although this chapter is devoted to partner support, the previous chapter connects the single mother with numerous other sources of support. You don't need a partner to have a successful breastfeeding experience, but you do need support.

### Educate yourself

Educate yourself about why breastfeeding, and especially breastfeeding in your special circumstance, is so important. Chapter 1, How Important Is It For You To Breastfeed?, will give you all the information that you need. When you understand why breastfeeding is so important, it will help you be more supportive of your partner and more committed to doing what it takes to make breastfeeding a success (Wolfberg et al., 2004).

Educate yourself about breastfeeding management: how to position and latch the baby, use a breast pump, hand express, store human milk, how often to breastfeed or express, and how to overcome common difficulties. A study by Pisacane et al. (2005) found that breastfeeding rates more than quadrupled for mothers who encountered breastfeeding problems when fathers were educated on breastfeeding management. This book will provide much of what you need to know. It probably isn't necessary for you to read it cover to cover, but if you familiarize yourself with all it has to offer, it can become an invaluable reference. I recommend that you and your partner have another general breastfeeding book to address breastfeeding issues not specifically related to breastfeeding without birthing. My website also has links to excellent online resources. One mother reported that when she was having difficulty latching her baby in the middle of the night, her husband brought his laptop into their bed and they watched an online breastfeeding demonstration. It was just what she needed that night to help her baby to latch (Tohotoa et al., 2009)!

**Accept the Commitment**

Breastfeeding requires an emotional commitment. At first, you can expect that breastfeeding without birthing will require a lot of effort. Parenting itself is a huge adjustment, and adding breastfeeding to the mix means even more new things to learn. Yet over time, you and your partner will figure out how to make it work for your family. When a woman induces lactation, she will also be adjusting to hormonal changes, since hormones drive milk production. I don't need to tell you that accepting hormonal changes in your partner requires emotional commitment! Be willing to hang in there with your partner.

Breastfeeding requires a time commitment for both you and your partner. Your partner will be breastfeeding and/or expressing her milk at least eight times per day. There may also be bottle-feeding, finger-feeding, and/or cup-feeding. Breastfeeding tools, such as breast pump parts and at-breast supplementers, must be cleaned routinely. Teaching an older or ill baby to breastfeed can be a lengthy process. Be willing to accept your partner's time commitment and give some of your own time as well. Be the official washer of breast-pump parts or preparer of the at-breast supplementer. *Be there* for your partner, whether that means sitting with her while she breastfeeds your baby, going with her to lactation consultations, or taking extra time off of work. One mother reported that she pumped more milk when her husband sat with her than when she pumped alone!

Breastfeeding also requires a financial commitment, but not breastfeeding requires a financial commitment too! In a typical breastfeeding situation, the costs of breastfeeding are minimal as compared to the costs of not breastfeeding: between $700 and $3,100 USD for formula for the first year (Bonyata, 2012), plus bottles and bottle nipples, additional doctor visits and prescriptions, and missed time from work due to a sick baby. Breastfeeding without birthing is harder to quantify because it requires additional breastfeeding support and supplies, and may also involve some costs of formula feeding.

## Jason's Story: Using His Talents

*When I was working with Kelly and Jason, who were expecting twins through surrogacy, Kelly was interested in supplementing the babies with the Lact-Aid at-breast supplementer. The Lact-Aid consists of a bag which hangs from a cord around mother's neck and is filled with expressed milk or formula. A feeding tube carries the milk or formula from the bag to the mother's nipple so she can provide extra food for him right there while breastfeeding. When I showed the couple how to assemble the Lact-Aid, Jason came alive. He was more adept with the device than I was. "Are you an engineer or something?" I asked. Sure enough, he was! What a great way for this father to use his talents to support his partner.*

## "To Protect and Defend"

Let this be your breastfeeding oath to your partner. Some friends, family members, co-workers, adoption/surrogacy/legal professionals, and even healthcare professionals may not be supportive of her decision to breastfeed. (See the sidebar, When Others Are Critical, in the previous chapter.) Protect and defend her against these naysayers. Tell them what a gift she is giving to your child and how proud you are of her. Help surround her with supportive people and help her to find professional help. There is a time and place even for supportive people, and your partner may need you to be a gatekeeper when she needs to nest in privacy.

## Nurture the Nurturer

Mothers nurture their babies through breastfeeding, and in many other ways, but constantly giving to her baby can leave a new mother depleted. You can take care of your partner so that she can take care of your baby through breastfeeding. Talk to your partner about how she needs to be nurtured. Make a list and review it over time as her needs change. Some ideas for caring for your breastfeeding partner include:

- **Anticipate her needs regarding food, sleep/rest, taking a shower, exercising, getting out of the house, or simply being alone.** Most parents are surprised how difficult it can sometimes be for a new mother to get these basic needs met.
- **Set up a nursing nook.** Partners can make sure the new mother has a comfortable and pleasant place to breastfeed or express her milk. The nursing nook includes a comfortable place to sit. Your partner may feel most comfortable in a private area, such as the nursery or your bedroom, or she may be happiest in a higher-traffic area, such as the living room. Nursing nooks often include a table for a healthy beverage, a book or magazine, TV remote control, or phone. Create a relaxing and enjoyable atmosphere for breastfeeding

or expressing milk: play music, light a candle, or turn on a good movie.

- **Respect her needs regarding touch.** Hormonal changes along with the intense physical needs of the baby can leave some new mothers feeling "touched out." Your partner may not want much physical affection from you, at least at first. For some mothers, breasts are off limits to her partner while she is breastfeeding. Or, she may especially appreciate your affections during this time. Touch can also help with breastfeeding. Any kind of touch, especially massage, while breastfeeding or expressing milk increases oxytocin levels. Oxytocin is the hormone that causes the milk to flow. Massage between the shoulder blades can be particularly helpful in releasing milk when mother is breastfeeding or using a breast pump.

### Be the Left to Her Right

You may have heard the term "baby brain" describing how a woman has difficulty following directions, thinking sequentially, processing information, and remembering facts when she is pregnant or has a new baby. Breastfeeding experts are beginning to understand that it is not that women's brains don't function as well when they have a new baby; it is that they become more right-brained. Dealing with facts, numbers, and instructions is left-brained functionality, whereas the right brain is wired for developing relationships, instincts, and intuition (Mohrbacher, 2010; Smillie, 2008). Nature has provided an excellent design because babies generally latch more easily and comfortably when breastfeeding is approached in a more instinctual and intuitive—right-brained—way. However, using left-brained skills, especially in special situations, such as breastfeeding without birthing, can provide the necessary balance of brain power for optimal breastfeeding outcomes.

I see this in my private practice all the time. New mothers have excellent instincts when it comes to breastfeeding, and it is my job to encourage them and offer some direction in following those instincts. Generally, though, new mothers with breastfeeding challenges are also in need of practical information. The only way I can expect them to keep track of this detailed information is to write it down for them in a breastfeeding-care plan. Even then, I suspect that they often forget to read the plan! This is where partners come in. You can keep track of all of the left-brained information, such as:

- The breastfeeding plan that you develop with the help of this book and an International Board Certified Lactation Consultant (IBCLC),
- Lists of local breastfeeding resources,
- Lists of helpful websites and books, and
- Important dates, such as doctor and lactation appointments, when mother started taking a medication or herb, and when her breast-pump rental fee is due.

You can also maintain the inventory of infant formula or donor breast milk; pumping supplies, such as storage bags; and feeding supplies, such as parts for an at-breast supplementer.

I have vivid memories calling my husband at work when our first baby was crying so intensely and I could not console him. I was overcome with emotions, but he could think logically. He had a mental list of the most simple, basic things to try in those situations. Most of the time, one of them worked! Even when they didn't, his calm voice of reason helped me to feel more balanced. You will, no doubt, have similar opportunities.

## Parent in a Way that Supports Attachment

This book has a whole chapter devoted to parenting tools (in addition to breastfeeding) that can help your baby attach to you and to his mother. I encourage you to read Chapter 6, Tools for Latching and Attaching, and see if you might be interested in practicing some of the parenting tools presented there: babywearing, co-sleeping, and co-bathing. These tools not only support attachment, they can also help your baby to learn to breastfeed.

That being said, your baby may need to attach first to his breastfeeding mother before he is ready to attach to a second parent. That was our family's experience with our adopted daughter, Rosa. For her first nine months or so, Rosa would become hysterical when she was held by anyone other than me. Then she added her father to the list. A few months later, she would permit other loving caregivers to hold her as well. At the time, I had a strong sense that she knew she had lost her first mother, and felt like she had to frantically protect her relationship with me. In this case, your role will be to support your partner's attachment parenting. Eventually, your turn will come.

## Practical Help

You can offer practical help with the baby and other household tasks, or arrange for outside help for some of these tasks: friends, family, housekeeper, a take-out restaurant, or a postpartum doula. Some areas to consider are:

- Diapering, bathing, and dressing baby
- Cooking
- Cleaning
- Washing breastfeeding and bottle-feeding supplies and tools, such as pump parts and the at-breast supplementer

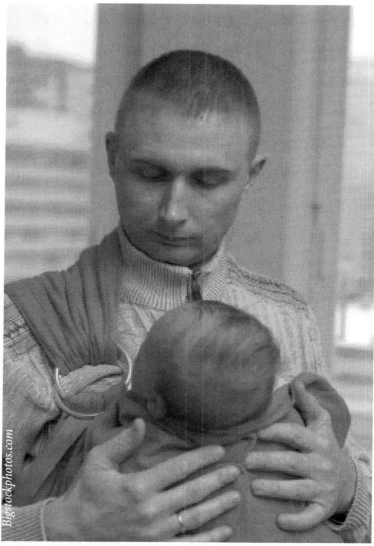

Father wearing his baby in a sling.

Breastfeeding without birthing may not be easy, but it is very worthwhile. There are so many ways you can support your partner's breastfeeding success, both with your attitude and your actions. Your support of breastfeeding is a lifelong gift you give your baby and your partner. It only *seems* like breastfeeding is a one-person job!

# Section II

# Latching—Nurturing at the Breast

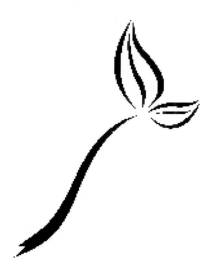

# Chapter 4

# LATCHING: WHAT TO EXPECT

Being able to latch your baby to the breast is half of the breast-feeding equation. (Making milk is the other half.) For some of your babies, learning to latch will be the same, or at least similar, to latching a baby who was born to you. For babies who begin breastfeeding from the get-go, latching onto the breast is imprinted, instinctual, and the only way of feeding the baby knows. These are healthy, full-term babies who are:

- Breastfed by the gestational mother, and go directly to breast-feeding by the breastfeeding-without-birthing mother, or
- Babies who are breastfed by their breastfeeding-without-birthing mother right from birth. This is generally the case with surrogacy. Mothers who are adopting babies at birth may or may not be able to, or may not choose to, breastfeed until adoption paperwork is signed by the birthmother.

Although some of these babies may still have some difficulty with latch, as babies sometimes do, the difficulties are more likely to be caused by issues not related to breastfeeding without birthing.

This chapter, and the remaining chapters in this section are dedicated to those adopted and foster babies who begin breastfeeding under less-than-optimal circumstances. These circumstances include babies who are not newborn, and those who are not healthy, either physically, emotionally, or developmentally. For these babies, the road to breastfeeding is likely to be long. In some cases, breastfeeding may never be achieved. It is impossible to predict how long or difficult it may be to get baby to latch at the breast. It all depends on where you and your baby are starting out.

## Factors in the Baby

### Age when Breastfeeding is Initiated

Babies who are less than eight weeks old are most likely to latch on without difficulty (Auerbach & Avery, 1981). Expect the process of learning to latch to take longer for an older baby, because the instincts for breastfeeding diminish over time. Even so, children as old as four years at placement have learned to breastfeed (Gribble, 2006).

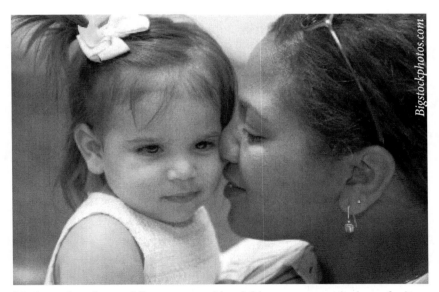

Mothers who adopt toddlers, or even older children, may consider breastfeeding.

## How Old is "Too Old" to Initiate Breastfeeding?

Our culture's support for breastfeeding tends to end when the baby turns a year of age. This cut-off may stem from the American Academy of Pediatrics, statement that babies should be breastfed for "at least the first year of life" (AAP, 2005). When evaluating this statement, I encourage you to consider this statement carefully. The statement does not suggest that babies be breastfed for one year, but for a *minimum* of one year. Studies that eliminate societal impacts have found that natural weaning for humans occurs between 2.5 and 7 years of age (Dettwyler, 2003). These findings are not terribly surprising considering the number of toddlers, and even preschoolers, who continue to use a bottle or a pacifier: modern substitutes for breastfeeding.

When considering whether your baby is too old to breast-feed, it is also important to consider that the emotional and developmental age of an adopted child is likely to be quite a bit younger than her biological age (Gribble, 2006).

### Prior Feeding Experience

If a baby has ever breastfed, that behavior is imprinted and may be retrieved by the adoptive, foster, or relactating mother. If a baby was bottle-fed while held close by a loving, consistent caregiver, the road to breastfeeding may still not be that long. However, if the baby was never held, her bottle was propped, and the nipple enlarged to speed up the feeding, learning to breastfed is likely to be a long and challenging process.

## Baby's Emotional Health

If a baby is coming to you from an institution or an abusive situation, she may find it extremely uncomfortable to receive eye contact or to be held, let alone to be able to achieve the intimate relationship of breastfeeding. While the journey to breastfeeding may be long for these precious babies, these are the babies who most need the emotional benefits it provides.

### Children Who Seek Breastfeeding

Some babies, toddlers, and even children as old as 12 years will seek to breastfeed from an adoptive or foster mother, whether or not the mother initiates the behavior. The child may attempt to remove mother's clothing, seek latching when skin-to-skin, or verbally ask to nurse. Children who seek breastfeeding may have been breastfed at one time. Or they may have never breastfed, but their newborn instincts have been re-awakened once they finally attach to their adoptive or foster mother in a safe, secure environment. The desire to breastfeed may even be triggered by the stress of the placement, as the child regresses into earlier behavior patterns. Regardless of the reason, if this is your experience, you are not alone (Gribble, 2005; 2006).

# Factors in the Mother

## Motivation

Perhaps the most critical factor in any mother's ability to latch her baby is her level of motivation. La Leche League leaders will often encourage mothers with the mantra: patience and persistence. As you will read in the following chapters, countless ideas are available for helping your baby latch at the breast. The mother who is ultimately able to breastfeed a difficult-to-latch baby is one who is ready to try different approaches, creative in finding solutions that work for her and her baby, willing to ask for help, and prepared to hang in there for the long run.

## Prior Breastfeeding Experience

A mother's prior breastfeeding experience goes a long way in helping her baby learn to breastfeed. A mother who has already breastfed has skills, confidence, and a support network built out of her past experience. She can draw from previous resources, and in some cases, may even have another nursling at home to help "teach" the new baby to breastfeed. Her breasts also have "prior experience" making milk, which is likely to result in more milk production, further encouraging the baby at the breast.

## Milk Production

Although this book addresses latching at the breast and milk production as two separate aspects of breastfeeding, they are in fact interdependent components of breastfeeding. When a mother produces more milk, suckling at the breast becomes a more satisfying experience for her baby. Babies, particularly those under one year of age (developmentally), are much more likely to be interested in suckling at the breast if the breast is producing milk. Swallowing mouthfuls of milk is positive reinforcement for good suckling.

Fortunately, if a mother is not producing milk, or not producing much milk, the flow of milk from the breast can be simulated using an at-breast supplementer, such as the Lact-Aid or Supplemental Nursing System (SNS). These devices, discussed in detail in Chapter 13, Supplementation, provide expressed milk or infant formula through a feeding tube at the mother's nipple so that the baby receives an ample flow from a breast with less-than-full milk production. They essentially serve as an external-milk-duct!

On the other hand, some mothers who produce very little milk successfully breastfeed their babies without an at-breast supplementer. They provide food for their baby in another way, usually a bottle. The baby suckles at the breast for comfort, much as many babies in our culture use a pacifier.

**Parenting Style**

Parenting style can greatly influence a baby's ability to latch at the breast. When parents are quick to respond to their baby's cues and keep their babies physically close to them, both during the day and at night, they are fostering strong communication between mother and baby, facilitating the learning process. Frequent body contact, especially skin-to-skin contact, puts the baby in the breastfeeding environment and awakens breastfeeding instincts in both the mother and the baby. The following chapters introduce some parenting tools that facilitate readiness and latching at the breast. (See Chapter 5, Honoring the Transition, and Chapter 6, Tools for Latching and Attaching.)

## Valuing the Process, Not Just the Product

When you have plenty of motivation and support, your baby has a good chance of learning to latch at the breast. But what if, despite your devoted efforts, your baby does not latch? Your efforts will not have been in vain. Any movement towards latching is incredibly valuable to your baby, and to your relationship with your baby. A baby who has never attached to a caregiver but learns to be cuddled, has come a great distance--even if she never latches at the breast. A baby who has a history of abuse, who now learns that her cries will be responded to, has learned trust--even if she never latches at the breast. The goal of these next few chapters is to meet your baby where she is and travel as far along the path to attachment and breastfeeding as is possible.

# Chapter 5

# HONORING THE TRANSITION

This chapter is about starting with your baby wherever he is and gently, respectfully bringing him to the point where he is ready to try breastfeeding. If your baby is a newborn, then he does not have a caregiving history outside the womb. He is probably ready to try breastfeeding. If your baby is older, however, he was cared for someone else before you. He will have to gradually transition to your loving, consistent care. Your baby will be ready to try breastfeeding when he is:

- Secure in your care,
- Able to make eye contact,
- Comfortable being held close to you, and
- Able to suckle from a slow-flow bottle nipple.

If your baby is able to do all of these things, feel free to proceed to the next chapter. Otherwise, this chapter is about getting your baby to this point where breastfeeding can be introduced.

# Honoring Your Baby's Transition

## Maintain Consistency

One way to ease the transition for an older baby is to maintain as much consistency as possible when he first arrives. Use familiar items whenever possible: clothing, blankets, diapers, soaps and lotions, toys, and especially bottles and formula. Think about all of the baby's senses: sight, sound, smell, touch, and taste. For instance, clothing and blankets should not be washed right away so that they will maintain their familiar smells (Caughman & Motley, 2009). Also, use routines that are familiar to him whenever possible and acceptable to you: sleeping, bathing, dressing, diapering, and feeding.

Because breastfeeding will likely be a new way of feeding your child, consider this transition carefully. Your internationally adopted baby in particular may have received bottles in a very different way than we know bottle-feeding in the United States. In order to save time in large institutions, where there are few caregivers for many babies, bottles may have been propped so that babies didn't need to be held during a feeding, and bottle nipples may have been enlarged to speed the feeding. The formula itself may have been quite different than what is available to you: it may be have been sweetened or had other substances added to it, such as coffee.

Lois Melina (1998), author of *Raising Adopted Children*, suggests that adoptive parents adjust bottle-feeding, at least at first, to mimic as close as reasonably possible the bottle-feeding experiences that babies received in their native countries. Over time, parents can gradually transition the baby, watching his cues for readiness, to bottle-feeding in a way that supports the eventual transition to breastfeeding: holding baby close while feeding, using the slowest flow bottle nipple, and filling the bottle with expressed human milk if available. Bottle-feeding strategies for transitioning from the bottle to the breast are discussed in Chapter 8, Additional Strategies for Latching.

## Minimize Stimulation

Another way that parents can honor the transition for the older baby is to limit stimulation. Because so many of the sensory inputs and routines cannot be maintained (and in many cases, should not be maintained), once baby is with his new family, new parents can limit the extent of new stimuli. Cocoon with your new baby for the first few weeks, if possible: don't leave the house with your baby and don't invite guests in. This may sound unkind to your loving extended family and friends, but it is a very short period of time for them to wait--and a very crucial period of time for your new baby. You can even keep your baby within a few rooms in your home and keep household noise, such as TV and music, to a minimum (although quiet soothing music may be helpful).

Minimizing stimulation can also refer to the physical stimulation from you. Your baby's senses may be over-stimulated because of a new environment and caregivers, prior abuse, or exposure to drugs or alcohol in utero. When your baby closes his eyes tightly, averts his gaze, splays his fingers, or fusses at your attentions, he may be communicating that he is overtired, overwhelmed, or over-stimulated. Your close physical presence without physical stimulation (talking, singing, touching) may be reassuring while respectful of your baby's needs. Or, you may find your baby benefits from certain types of sensory input from you.

Skin-to-skin contact with mother is the most organizing input for most infants. Some infants respond to rhythmic rocking or swaying while held snuggled firmly against an adult's chest, gentle swinging from head to toe in a gathered up blanket or swaddling with the hands placed near the face. Some infants respond to repetitive sounds, such as the traditional shushing sound, during these vestibular/tactile stimulation activities. Sucking is organizing for infants, and brief non-nutritive sucking on an adult finger (with appropriate infection control practices) or a pacifier/dummy may be used to help an infant achieve an organized state. Hunger can be disorganizing for infants, and giving a small amount of milk in a way that is workable for the infant (spoon, cup, finger feeding, bottle) may allow the baby to settle and work at breastfeeding (Genna, 2008, pp. 240-241).

If your baby continues to have difficulty processing sensory inputs, consult with an occupational therapist that specializes in sensory integration.

## Understand your Baby's Need to Grieve

An essential aspect of healing for your baby is grieving the loss of his first attachment(s). As your baby gradually connects with you, he will need to release the pain of his broken attachments. You may observe this release in the following behavior: he may cry, rest, and then be ready to connect further (Lee, 2011). The parenting tools introduced in the next chapter provide rich opportunities for you to comfort your child while he grieves. They are comforting and reassuring to your child and provide a safe, secure environment for your baby to grieve.

Talking with your baby may help too. Even babies who are too young to understand your words can tune into your emotions. Talk to your baby about his history, tell him how sorry you are for the pain and loss he has experienced, and tell him you love him and will always be there for him. Empty your heart to him. Tell him about your hopes for breastfeeding, and how it will help him grow strong and healthy, both physically and emotionally. Talking in soothing tones will help your baby to heal, will help you to heal, and will help the two of you to connect with each other.

Therapy may also be available to help your child heal from early loss, abuse, or neglect. CranioSacral therapy is a type of gentle, non-invasive bodywork that has been very effective at helping babies connect with their mothers, breastfeed more comfortably and effectively, sleep better, and experience less pain (Lee, 2011). To learn more about CranioSacral therapy and to find CranioSacral therapist in your area, see *www.upledger.com*. Your local lactation consultant in private practice may also be able to refer you to a practitioner trained and experienced with babies.

## Bethany's Story: Mother and Daughter Connect

*When Bethany brought six-month-old Linn home from Korea, transitioning from bottle-feeding to breastfeeding was "definitely a process." Linn was constantly testing Bethany: will you be there for me? Bethany knew that she needed to build trust before breastfeeding would be possible. At one point, after a gut-wrenching cry, Linn started "talking" to Bethany. Bethany believes Linn was telling her story to her adoptive mother. That day was a turning point in their relationship: it was when they finally felt like mother and daughter.*

## Honoring Your Transition

This chapter up to this point has been devoted to helping your new baby attach to you. It is also important to recognize that, as adoptive, intended, or foster mothers, attaching to your baby may also be difficult for you. Gestational mothers have nine months of watching their abdomen grow and feeling the physical changes of pregnancy in which to begin bonding to their new baby. You cannot expect yourself to connect with your brand-new little person on the spot. Furthermore, many of you have waited a long time and endured a lot of heartache to get to this point. You may have built up walls protecting your emotions from yet another disappointment. Even when your baby is in arms, it can take some time for the walls to come down, and for you to feel safe falling in love with your child. Give yourself time and space to adjust to being your new baby's parent (Sember, 2007). Attachment is a process that both you and your child will go through. Fortunately, time and the parenting tools in the next chapter not only help your little one attach to you, they also help you attach to your little one.

# Chapter 6

# TOOLS FOR LATCHING AND ATTACHING

Breastfeeding is just one parenting tool that promotes attachment to your baby. This chapter introduces other some parenting tools that facilitate attachment[1]— and, as an added bonus, they can help your baby learn to breastfeed. Chapter 4, Latching: What to Expect, described how some babies and young children will seek breastfeeding from their adoptive mother who did not intend to breastfeed. In many of the situations reported in the research literature, the child sought to breastfeed when the adoptive mother was practicing one of these parenting tools (Gribble, 2005). Mothers who intend to breastfeed can also use the tools to connect with their baby, and to awaken the instincts to breastfeed in their child and in themselves. Using these tools can:

- **Reset your baby's start in life**. Experiences that remind baby of her time in the womb can essentially reprogram her start in life when her instincts to breastfeed were at their peak.

- **Offer your baby opportunities to breastfeed by placing her**

---

[1]The tools presented in this chapter are appropriate for a baby who is comfortable being held close, skin-to-skin, with eye contact. If your baby isn't ready for these things, refer back to the previous chapter, Honoring the Transition, and then proceed to these tools gently, cautiously, and, if needed, persistently.

**close to your breasts**. These parenting practices mean that baby is in the breastfeeding environment, often skin-to-skin, associating warmth, security, and comfort with mother's chest, and encouraging her to give breastfeeding a try.

- **Cultivate trust in your baby that you will respond sensitively to her signals.** These signals include letting you know that she needs to be fed and nurtured, needs that are both satisfied so well with breastfeeding. These parenting tools help you to be in tune with your baby's cues, facilitating communication between the two of you as you are teaching her to nurse.

Although breastfeeding is exclusive to mothers, all of the tools presented below for latching and attaching can be practiced by both parents. Yes, the baby's instincts to nurse can be stimulated by the non-breastfeeding partner. No problem. This just means it is time for a hasty hand-off to mother! By practicing these tools, the partner is attaching to his or her baby while at the same time supporting breastfeeding.

The tools of latching and attaching are babywearing, co-sleeping, and co-bathing. Some of these tools will fit your personality and lifestyle better than others. I encourage you to be open to considering new ideas. I remember saying that co-sleeping was just fine for other mothers and babies, but I would NEVER do that with my baby. Can you guess that I ended up loving co-sleeping with all of my babies? Try them out and use whichever tools feel right for you and your baby. The tools that work for you may be different than what works best for your partner. You will find a set of tools that work for your family. Be ready for them to change over time as you, your partner, and your baby grow in your family together.

**Oxytocin, the Attachment Hormone**

Breastfeeding, babywearing, co-sleeping, and co-bathing are all tools of attachment. Did you know that there is also a hormone of attachment? Oxytocin is calming, and it enhances feelings of connection between mother and baby (Moberg, 2003). Whenever a mother and baby are in close body contact when using any of the tools for latching and attaching--especially when mother and baby are in skin-to-skin contact--levels of the hormone oxytocin increase in both mother and baby. And because oxytocin is also the hormone responsible for milk ejection, using the tools of latching and attaching supports a mother's ability to make milk, as well as her baby's ability to latch.

## Babywearing

Babywearing refers to carrying your baby in a soft baby carrier that provides direct body contact between you and your baby, and supports your baby's weight in much the same way you would hold your baby if you were to hold her in your arms: by her thighs and bottom. These types of baby carriers include the sling, pouch, *mei tai*, wrap, or backpack style (which can be worn on front or back).[2] The right type of carrier for you may depend on the size of your baby, your comfort and convenience, and whether you wish to breastfeed while babywearing (yes, it is possible and convenient, and a discreet way to breastfeed in public). You may find that you enjoy owning more than one type of carrier. My husband liked having his own!

---

[2] Be wary of other popular types of soft baby carriers. These carriers may have a layer of material between the baby and the adult, which limits the close body contact between you and your baby. These types of carriers generally also support your baby between her legs, which can cause hip dysplasia.

Babywearing can take some skill and practice. It can really help to have some other babywearing mothers around to observe and to help you if you need it. Search online for babywearing and your city's name: many cities have local babywearing groups or classes.

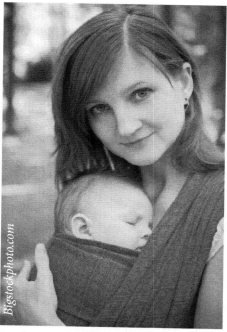

Mother is wearing her baby in a wrap.

## Babywearing Resets your Baby's Start in Life

Babywearing is a "womb with a view" (Granju & Kennedy, 1999). It is much like a baby's experience in utero: baby is snug and secure against her mother's body, hearing her heartbeat, smelling her scent (yes, babies can smell the amniotic fluid), and traveling in rhythm with her gait. One mother shared her babywearing experience in, *You Can Adopt: An Adoptive Families Guide.*

When I adopted my youngest daughter domestically, attachment was difficult because she was hospitalized for three months. When she came home, I bought a soft-sling baby carrier. It allowed me to hold her close to my heart in a comforting fetal position for much of the day. Not only did this improve our attachment, it improved her health immensely (Caughman & Motley, 2009, p. 201).

This incredible tool not only helps your baby connect with you as if in utero, it is an opportunity for you to feel pregnant with your baby. As a mother who has experienced pregnancy and babywearing, I can attest that babywearing (especially a newborn) feels very much like pregnancy. Have you seen pregnant women affectionately caressing their bellies? You may find the same instinct while wearing your baby, and it feels beautiful!

## Babywearing Offers Your Baby Opportunities to Breastfeed by Placing Her Close To Your Breasts

Consider how much closer your baby is to you when you are wearing her than when she is placed in or is transported in a stroller, car seat[3], bouncy seat, swing, or crib. Baby is in direct body contact with her mother, usually with her head close to mother's breast. Fathers, and mothers when in private, can even wear their babies skin-to-skin. Your baby is right there in the breastfeeding environment, calmed by the gentle rocking movement as you walk: a perfect opportunity for initiating breastfeeding.

---

[3]Babywearing is not appropriate while driving or performing other activities where your baby's safety would be compromised.

**Babywearing Cultivates Trust in Your Baby that You Will Respond Sensitively to Her Signals**

When a mother wears her baby, her communication with her baby is enhanced. She senses her baby's needs more quickly when she feels her baby's subtle movements against her body, observes her delicate facial expressions, and hears the small sounds that preempt her cries.

# Co-Sleeping

Co-sleeping is a very general term we will define as sleeping in close proximity to your baby. For many parents, sleeping in close proximity means sleeping with their baby in their bed. Other parents find that a co-sleeper or a crib attached to their bed in a sidecar arrangement works best. For other parents, the baby is in a separate bed within the parents' room. I encourage you to find the closest arrangement that works for you. For more information on co-sleeping, some excellent books are listed in Library page of my website.

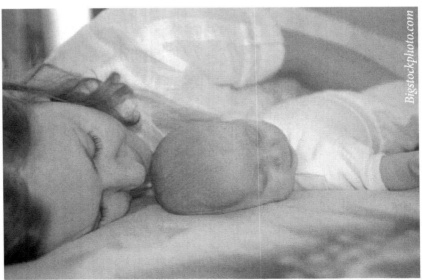

Mother and baby co-sleeping.

### Co-Sleeping Resets Your Baby's Start in Life

When a baby sleeps in utero, she is enveloped by her mother's body, surrounded by her warmth, smelling her amniotic fluid, and hearing her mother's heartbeat. When a baby co-sleeps with her mother, she is enveloped by her body, surrounded by her warmth, smelling her scent, and hearing her breathe. Co-sleeping can be a safe, secure, and comfortable cocoon we can create for our baby much like the cocoon of the womb.

### Co-Sleeping Offers Your Baby Opportunities to Breastfeed by Placing Her Close to Your Breasts

When your baby sleeps close to you, especially if you sleep bare-breasted, your baby is in the breastfeeding environment all night. She can smell the scent of your milk, if you are producing some. When your baby is drowsy or in a light sleep, her instincts to breastfeed are more easily aroused. When a mother is drowsy, she tends to behave more instinctively as well. Even when your baby does not show interest in latching, she is associating feelings of warmth and comfort with being close to your breast.

### Co-Sleeping Cultivates Trust in Your Baby that You Will Respond Sensitively to Her Signals

Parents who sleep in close proximity to their babies can respond to their nighttime needs more quickly, because they notice them sooner. Often, babies don't fully awaken before their parents respond and tend to their needs, including their needs to be fed and comforted.

## Co-Sleeping Safely with your Baby

Dr. James McKenna, Professor of Biological Anthropology and director of the Mother-Baby Sleep Laboratory at the University of Notre Dame, recommends these guidelines for safe mother-baby co-sleeping (McKenna, 2012).

- Baby should sleep on her back.
- Baby should sleep on a firm surface, with only a light blanket. The baby's head should not be covered.
- Baby should not have pillows or stuffed animals around her.
- Baby should never sleep alone, with a parent, or with some other person on a surface, such as a couch, that contains a crevice that the baby could fall into face-first.
- If your baby is not yet breastfeeding, the baby should sleep on a separate surface, either attached to or close by the parents' bed. Only breastfeeding babies can safely share a bed with their parents.
- Babies younger than a year should not share a bed with older siblings.
- Mothers with excessively long hair should tie their hair back, as very long hair could possibly strangle a baby.
- Parents should not bedshare when they are intoxicated, using sedatives, or otherwise slow to arouse.
- Parents should not smoke.

For more information, a link to Dr. McKenna's website can be found on the Links page of my website.

### My Story: The Outer Womb

*For her first nine months, Rosa lived almost 24 hours a day with me in her outer womb. She slept in bed with me at night. I carried her in a sling when I was awake, and fed her very frequently. When I was not doing these things, she cried. When her father or anyone else tried to hold her even for a couple of minutes, she cried. When I put her down to sleep in her cradle, she slept for five minutes, and then cried. Was it any coincidence that she needed nine months in my (outer) womb?*

# Co-Bathing

Co-bathing is simply taking a bath with your baby. Gently recline in the bathtub and place your baby tummy down on your chest. Your breasts should be above the water line so that they are available in case your baby is interested in nursing. Since you and your baby will only be partially immersed, keep both you and your baby warm by maintaining a warm temperature in the bathroom and frequently pouring warm bathwater over your baby's back (Lee, 2011). Co-bathing can be easy, relaxing, and enjoyable for you and your baby. It can also be a great way to encourage a baby to breastfeed.

### Co-Bathing Resets Your Baby's Start in Life

When you take a bath with your baby, it takes your baby back to her time in utero … this time around with you enveloping her in the warm, watery, bathtub womb! You can further simulate the womb environment by minimizing light: turn off the bathroom light and use only candlelight or the light from the hallway.

Co-bathing is such an extremely powerful reminder of the time in the womb, that lactation consultant Nikki Lee (2011) warns the co-bathing mother that her baby may work through events from her past when she revisits this time in the womb: her baby may crawl toward the breast, cry a little, then continue toward the breast, repeating the process several times.

## Co-Bathing Offers Your Baby Opportunities to Breastfeed by Placing Her Close to Your Breasts

With both of you naked, baby's head on your chest, how much closer can you get than this?

## Co-Bathing Cultivates Trust in Your Baby that You Will Respond Sensitively to Her Signals

In the bathtub with your baby, you may feel as if you have created a little world of just the two of you. Within the confines of the tub, there is little to distract you from every nuance of your baby's sounds and movements. Responding to her communication with your own builds a foundation of trust.

# Chapter 7

# FINALLY...LATCHING!

*When nothing seems to help, I go and look at a stone-cutter hammering away at his rock perhaps a hundred times without as much as a crack showing in it. Yet at the hundred and first blow it will split in two, and I know it was not that blow that did it, but all that had gone before.*

- Jacob Riis

Your baby is ready to learn to latch onto your breast, receiving nourishment and nurturing from breastfeeding. He may have been ready from the moment the two of you met, or you might have been working with him for a while to get to this point by "honoring the transition," as described in Chapter 5. Practicing the parenting tools for latching and attaching from the previous chapter sets the foundation for breastfeeding. But how do you start?

This chapter will provide you with the tools and techniques to help your baby to breastfeed, and to awaken your own breastfeeding instincts as a mother. All of the suggestions for helping your baby to latch are intended to gently guide your baby towards breastfeeding. No pressure. Instead, be patient with yourself and your baby. Know that every attempt at breastfeeding is a success because you have bonded with your baby in the process and moved one step closer to your goal.

# Calm Surroundings

Before you attempt to latch your baby onto your breast, set the stage for success. The goal is to create a calm, gentle, and loving environment for you and your baby.

How do you like to get comfortable and unwind? When you are relaxed, you will be more in touch your mothering instincts, and you will enjoy this special time with your baby more. Because your baby is connected to you, he will be more relaxed when you are relaxed. Creating calm for your baby will help him further connect with you and be more instinctive. Some things that can you can do in your environment that can create calm for you and/or your baby are:

- **A Darkened Room**. When the room is dim, there is less stimulation and distraction for both you and your baby. Allow you and your baby to be the entire universe during this special time.
- **Candlelight**. Candlelight provides soft lighting and a sense of warmth. You may not wish to choose scented candles, even though they are very pleasant and relaxing. We don't want anything to get in the way of your baby connecting with your smell.
- **Soft Music.** Soft music can be relaxing. Or, try nature sounds that include flowing water to stimulate some flowing of your own!

- **Remove or use distractions, whichever you find most helpful**. You may find distractions, such as television and phone, take your focus away from your baby and make it more difficult to practice latching. On the contrary, you may find hands-free distractions, such as watching television or talking with a friend or loved one, can take away some of the pressure to get baby latched and give you more patience with the process. Whatever works for you is the right choice.

- **Only offer the breast if your baby is in a calm—even drowsy—state**. If the day has been very stimulating, if he isn't feeling well, or he needs a new diaper, it may not be the best time for your baby to learn a new skill.

Your baby will feel most calm skin to skin with you, and not-at-all calm if he is hungry.

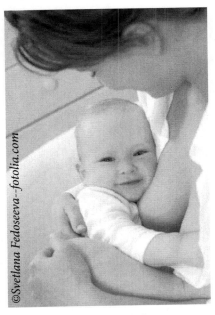

©Svetlana Fedoseeva–fotolia.com

Help your baby to latch by creating a positive association for your baby with being at the breast.

# Skin to Skin

Before even offering the breast, calm your baby and yourself by placing him skin to skin against your chest. Skin to skin means your baby is naked except for his diaper, and you are bare from the waist up.

Your baby touches your skin with his, breathes in your scent, and hears the steady rhythm of your heart. You enjoy his soft skin and hair against your bare chest, and sense every nuance of his movements and sweet baby sounds. If your baby or you are chilly, place a blanket over both of you, or you can wear a large bathrobe and wrap it around both of you. When you are skin to skin this way, your baby has a positive association with being in the breastfeeding habitat.

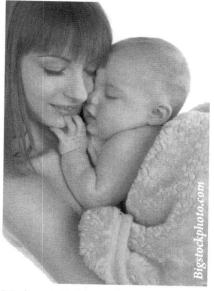

Mother and baby are skin to skin with a blanket wrapped around the two of them for warmth.

## When Your Baby Is Not Comfortable Skin to Skin

But what if skin to skin does just the opposite of calming your baby? For various reasons, some babies can become upset when they are skin to skin against their mothers' chest. If this happens with your baby, you will need to spend some time creating a positive association with skin to skin before your baby is ready to latch onto the breast. He must be comfortable and happy, with his little face next to your bare breasts: breastfeeding mother and blogger Stephanie Cornais suggests that you "make your boobs a happy place." She came up with some amazing ways to use play to help her daughter Penelope become comfortable skin to skin against her breasts and ready to breastfeed.

> Once I realized I needed to get Penelope to have a positive association first and foremost, I stopped actively trying to get Penelope to latch and I focused on ... play[ing] games with her at the breast and giv[ing] her lots of positive reinforcement. I would hold her in a cradle position with my boob out and her head resting on my boob or just being nearby. Then I would hold my boob so that my nipple was kind of tickling her cheek or mouth and smile big and say, "Yay! Penelope!" Or I would have a clutching toy for her to look at while I had her in a cradle or side lying position, and we would just play "in position," and that helped let her guard down about being "in position." I would also use the toy to get her to turn her head towards my nipple. When she did turn her head towards me I would say, "Yay! Penelope!" Before I could get her to be held in a cradle position, I would do this laying down next to her, or sometimes even on top of her on all fours, and let my boobs just kind of dangle, and I would sing songs and smile. I would do anything I could think of, to make her smile while my boob was nearby. (Make your boobs a happy place, 2010)

To read more about Penelope's journey to breastfeeding, you can find the rest of Stephanie's blog post at *mamaandbabylove. com/2010/12/31/make-your-boobs-a-happy-place/*.

# Not (Too) Hungry

One way to very quickly frustrate your baby can be to try to teach him to breastfeed when he is really hungry. Would you do well learning a new skill on an empty stomach, or would you learn better if you had been comfortably fed beforehand? It is the same for your baby, even though the new skill he is learning is how to eat. Most babies start breastfeeding without needing to drink a lot of milk. Consider a newborn baby nursing from his gestational mother: her mature milk doesn't come in until a few days after birth; before then, baby is learning to breastfeed from breasts producing very small quantities of colostrum. Your baby will also benefit from nursing for practice and comfort, at first. If you offer the breast when your baby is not too hungry, it also takes a little pressure off of you getting your baby fed.

On the other hand, your baby may not be motivated to take the breast if he is too satisfied from a bottle or pacifier. He may be much more interested in taking a nap, observing the world around him, or playing!

There are several ways to offer your baby the breast when he is not too hungry but not too full.

- **Bottle-feed your baby at the breast.** Bottle-feeding at the breast helps transition your baby to breastfeeding and associates a comfortably full tummy with the breast. Feed your baby with his cheek resting against your bare breast, essentially bottle-feeding in as close to the breastfeeding position as possible. When your baby is feeling content, but not completely full, offer the "breast for dessert." If your baby has his cheek resting on your breast, he is already sitting at the restaurant ready for the next course! It is a matter of deftly removing the bottle and shifting baby's position slightly so that his torso is facing you. Baby is now in a breastfeeding position. This technique is sometimes called the "bait and switch."

- **Finger-feed your baby first**. Finger-feeding is an infant feeding method in which the baby suckles on the caregiver's finger and receives expressed milk or formula through a tiny feeding tube resting on the finger. Because baby suckles on the finger in much the same way as he suckles on the breast, finger-feeding can start to fill baby's tummy, while at the same time help baby practice good breastfeeding technique. The feeding tube can even be transitioned from the finger to the breast when the breast is offered. See Chapter 13, Supplementation, for more information on finger-feeding and using a feeding tube at the breast.

- **Eliminate the pacifier.** Some mothers will not use a pacifier, and will offer the breast when her baby wants to suckle for comfort.

## Offer the Breast

The phrase "*offer* the breast" is used very deliberately throughout this chapter. Breastfeeding cannot be forced. Pushing your baby, and yourself, too hard can only create frustration for both of you, and it could even lead to your baby's aversion to the breast. Margaret Wills, IBCLC, suggests that every effort a mother makes towards breastfeeding is a success when a mother responds sensitively to her baby.

> If [mother] backs off if the baby seems a little frustrated, she lets the baby know that he/she is listened to. As long as we don't push the baby, there's no

down-side to her efforts--it's all good. [The mother] needs to feel that, even if the baby didn't latch that day, she didn't waste her efforts. (personal communication, February 10, 2012)

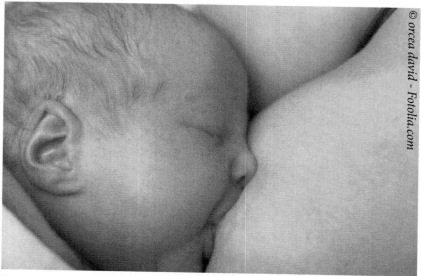

Baby is latched well: She is close to her mother, and has a wide gape.

Some persistence over time may be necessary before your baby latches. Learning to breastfeed is a process. Baby often starts first by licking the nipple, then suckling just a few times, and finally latching for several minutes. At first, short, frequent feeds may be easier for your baby. Provide lots of praise for any of the steps towards breastfeeding!

## Positioning for Learning to Breastfeed

Babies can breastfeed in a variety of positions. The most common breastfeeding position is the cradle hold, yet many mothers and babies find that other positions can be more helpful when getting started with breastfeeding. The key to success with all of these positions is that baby is stable, supported, and close to his mother (Genna, 2011).

## Cradle Hold

Most images of mothers who are breastfeeding show them positioning their baby in a cradle hold: baby is cradled in his mother's arm and nurses from the breast on that side. This tried-and-true position tends to be the preferred position of experienced mothers and babies. But what about babies who are learning to nurse, especially those who are learning to nurse when they are older? This position may be a good place to

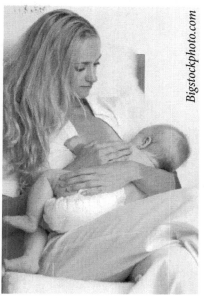

Cradle hold is the most common breastfeeding position.

start. If your baby has been bottle-feeding, he is probably accustomed to feeding in this position. In this case, it is a matter of turning your baby's body so that his torso is facing you, his tummy directly against your tummy, while his cheek continues to rest on your bare breast. When baby is first learning to breastfeed, you may or may not need to support your breast with your opposite hand.

Although the cradle hold is the most common breastfeeding position over the long run, several other positions are more commonly used with babies who are first learning to breastfeed. These may be helpful to try as well.

## Cross-Cradle Hold

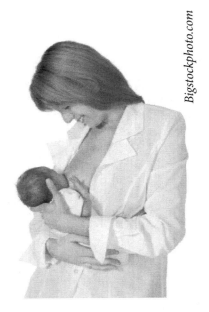

*Bigstockphoto.com*

The cross-cradle hold is similar to the cradle hold, except that the baby is held by the arm opposite the breast he is nursing from. This hold provides mother with a good bit of control over her baby's position, which is why it is a popular way new mothers and babies learn to breastfeed. Many mothers use a pillow to support their baby lying horizontally across their chest. The baby's body is supported by the mother's forearm, and possibly the pillow; the baby's head is cra-

This mother is supporting her baby with the opposite arm in the cross-cradle hold.

dled by mother's hand at the base of the skull, with her thumb on top and the remaining fingers below. Mother's other hand holds the same-sided breast with her thumb and other fingers in a U-shape. When baby's mouth is open wide, mother uses her forearm to pull baby close. Mother can tickle her baby's lips with her nipple or rest her nipple against the baby's philtrum (the indent between the nose and upper lip) to encourage her baby to open with a wide gape.

## Laid-Back Breastfeeding

Biological Nurturing™, or laid-back breastfeeding, is a great way to get breastfeeding off to a good start. British midwife Suzanne Colson discovered that when the mother is semi-reclined with her baby lying on his tummy on top of the mother's body, his body is fully supported by his mother's torso or surrounding furniture or pillows. This semi-reclined position, with the baby on top of the mother's body, releases the baby's and mother's inborn feeding behaviors. Mother's hand may be on her baby to offer some guidance and make sure that baby doesn't slide off her chest, but her hand does not support her baby's weight. Mother may hold her breast or she may not. Laid-back breastfeeding is a natural pairing of mother's natural instincts and the baby's inborn reflexes. While other positions typically use three inborn reflexes, laid-back breastfeeding has been associated with 20 inborn reflexes. With the help of all of these reflexes, babies can usually self-attach, resulting in a more comfortable and effective latch than when mothers initiate latching their babies (Colson, 2010).

Even if your baby is not a newborn, laid-back positioning can reset your baby, especially when done in skin to skin or while co-bathing.

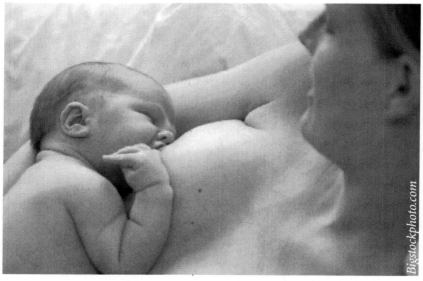

Laid-back breastfeeding is very relaxing for mother since she is semi-reclined and her whole body is supported. Laid-back breastfeeding helps baby to learn to latch using all of his newborn instincts for breastfeeding.

In the tub together, allow your baby to rest partially immersed with his tummy on your torso, cheek on your chest. If he begins to root, then follow his lead. (See Chapter 6, Tools for Latching and Attaching, for more information on co-bathing.)

Laid-back breastfeeding can also work very well when your baby is in a light sleep or in a drowsy state, lying on your chest with his sweet cheek on your breast (Colson, 2012).

### Side-Lying

I usually tell new mothers that the side-lying position is an "advanced breastfeeding technique." I encourage them to wait until breastfeeding is going smoothly in other positions before trying this position because it offers both mother and baby less control of the baby's position. However, if you are teaching an older baby to breastfeed, this position may be helpful, especially if you are co-sleeping with your baby. Your baby's instincts are more available when he is drowsy or in a light sleep, and so offering the breast while lying next to your baby, both of you on your side facing each other, might be the perfect timing. Sleeping enveloped by your scent will awaken your baby's breastfeeding instincts. Sleeping bare chested provides skin-to-skin contact and easy access. Tickle your baby's lips with your nipple when he is in a light-sleep stage, or just waking up, and see if he takes the bait!

### Nursing in Motion

Some babies are more likely to accept the breast when they are moving. Rhythmic movement is soothing and organizing for your baby. It is also reminiscent of baby's experience in the womb, which can help to reset your baby's breastfeeding instincts. Try offering the breast while wearing your baby in a soft baby carrier that provides direct contact between your baby and your chest. Your baby may be in the carrier a cradle position, or he may be front-facing. It can be easier to breastfeed in certain types of baby carriers than others. (See Chapter 6, Tools for Latching and Attaching, for more information on babywearing.) Offering the breast with the gentle movement of a rocking chair or glider can also be helpful for some babies.

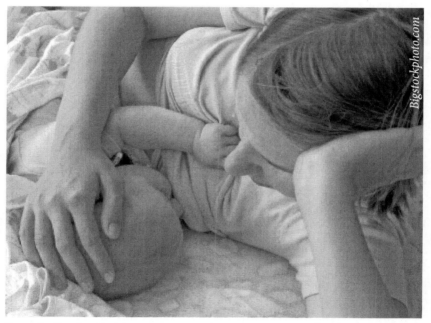

Breastfeeding in side-lying position can happen quite naturally when mother and baby are resting or sleeping close to each other.

## Offer Breast in a Totally Different Way

When traditional breastfeeding techniques aren't working for you and your baby, a creative approach might offer a fresh perspective for both of you. Consider this approach suggested by Catherine Watson Genna, IBCLC:

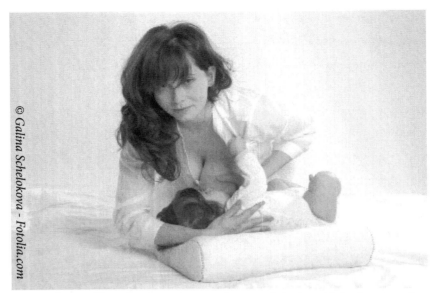

This mother is offering her breast in a creative way: baby is on his back and mother is leaning over him.

One three-month-old was happy to nurse after a tickle-with-nipple session. He cried when he saw mom's breast, so I had her lay him on his back on her bed, and had her try tickling his tummy with her nipple while making a silly sound (buzz!), then tickling his chest, his cheek, all the time getting closer to his mouth. When she tickled his philtrum (the little ridge between mouth and nose), he opened wide (it's a reflex) and she dropped in from the sky. He sucked, got milk, and nursed normally the next feeding! (personal communication, October 26, 2011)

## When You Are Not Producing Much Milk

When your baby latches onto the breast, he may expect a reward for his efforts: some delicious milk pouring into his mouth. If you are producing a significant quantity of milk, a few good suckles from your baby will give him just the reward he is looking for. But what if you aren't making much, or any, milk? It really depends on your baby whether the comfort from suckling at your breast will be enough to keep him interested. Many babies less than a year of age will require milk flowing from the breast to stay interested. If yours is one of those babies, and you are not (or not yet) producing much milk, you can add "an external milk duct" by delivering expressed milk or infant formula to your baby at your breast using a feeding tube attached to the breast. See Chapter 13, Supplementation, for more information on supplementing at the breast.

If you find the strategies presented in this chapter, together with patience and practice, are not enough to help your baby to the breast, the following chapter provides even more ideas to help.

# Chapter 8

# ADDITIONAL STRATEGIES FOR LATCHING

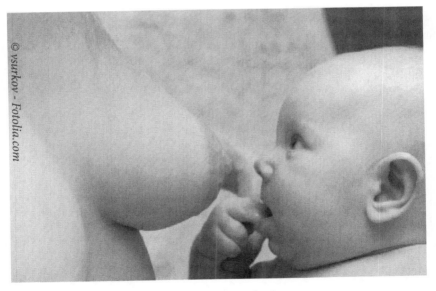

Some babies need a little extra help learning to latch.

For some babies, the basic strategies presented in the previous chapter for learning to latch onto the breast are not enough. This chapter provides some additional techniques that you may find helpful. Many ideas are presented here--my intention is not for you to try them all, but to use this as a menu of possibilities. Pick a few that feel right to you, and if those don't work, go back to the list. If you try something today that doesn't work, it may work later on.

If you are reading this chapter because you have not had success with the basic strategies in the last chapter for teaching your baby to breastfeed, I suggest that you contact an International Board Certified Lactation Consultant (IBCLC), if you haven't already done so. A lactation consultant can help with latching in two ways. First, she can help you put the latching techniques into action. Some of the techniques presented in this chapter, and the previous one, are simple. When trying other techniques, seeking the expertise and experience of a lactation consultant may be very helpful. Don't let yourself become frustrated with any of these strategies--help is available. The other reason to contact a lactation consultant is that the cause of your baby's difficulty with latching may be unrelated to breastfeeding without birthing. That was my experience: Rosa was born with a tongue-tie that was diagnosed when I received help from a lactation consultant.

## Model Breastfeeding

Do mothers and babies learn to breastfeed by instinct or by example? Recent research by Suzanne Colson (2010) has indicated that breastfeeding is instinctual for both mother and baby. However, it can be difficult to feel confident in this "natural" process that neither mother (in some cases) nor baby has ever seen or experienced before. Kirsten Berggren, Ph.D., IBCLC offers an excellent analogy with riding a bicycle.

> Think about your exposure to bicycles before you ever rode one. You probably saw them just about every day, your parents rode bikes at least once in a

while, and you wanted to learn so you could get out with the other kids in the neighborhood (who you saw every day). You had a certain knowledge of what riding a bike would look like before you even tried. Let's wander back to life 100 years ago--breastfeeding was like that. Families were larger, and most babies were born at home. That meant that from your earliest consciousness, you were exposed to breastfeeding. You saw your siblings or nieces and nephews breastfed. You watched breastfeeding with the boldness of a child—you put your head right by the mother's breast, you watched the baby's mouth, you absorbed breastfeeding into your knowledge of how the world worked (Berggren, 2009).

We don't live in a breastfeeding culture anymore, but you can invite breastfeeding into your life by showing your little one (and yourself) models of other babies or toddlers nursing.

## Ain't Nothin' Like The Real Thing, Baby!

There's nothing like seeing and being around real, live breastfeeding mothers and babies to encourage both mother and baby to breastfeed. If the breastfeeding mother is someone very close to you, you may have an opportunity to view breastfeeding up close. Even being in the same room as another breastfeeding mother provides information about how breastfeeding works and encouragement that it can work very well. It can also provide a boost of the hormone oxytocin, awakening your breastfeeding and nurturing instincts (Moberg, 2003). Check out this amazing true story about a fellow primate, a gorilla in the Columbus, Ohio zoo.

> The gorilla was born in captivity and was not part of a community of gorillas, so she had never seen another gorilla breastfeed. When she gave birth to her first gorilla baby, she had no idea how to feed her and the baby eventually died. When she became pregnant a second time, the zookeepers had an idea. They invited nursing mothers from the local La Leche League group, a mother-to-mother breastfeeding organization, to sit near the mother's cage and breastfeed their babies. After watching the human mothers breastfeed, the gorilla mother successfully breastfed her second gorilla baby (Mohrbacher & Kendall-Tackett, 2005, p. 17).

In Chapter 2, A Community of Support, we discussed building your support network, and this is one reason why: to provide opportunities to be around breastfeeding mothers and babies.

## Anne's Story: Surrounded by Breastfeeding Mothers and Babies

*Anne adopted Minh from Vietnam when he was about a year old. Although she tried over and over again, Anne was not able to latch Minh. Anne was disappointed that she would not be able to nurture her baby at the breast as she had her biological children, but she also knew of many other ways to attach to her baby. One of her favorites was carrying Minh in a sling. The sling proved very handy as Anne toted 18-month-old Minh around a La Leche League conference for three days. Minh spent three days carried close to his mother's breast surrounded by countless breastfeeding babies. To his mother's surprise and amazement, at the end*

106

*of the three days, Minh spontaneously latched onto his mother's breast for the first time! After that, Minh was a breastfeeding baby.*

When live breastfeeding mothers aren't available, you can still introduce images of breastfeeding to you and your baby. In some of these cases, looking at breastfeeding up close may be more accessible when you are not observing a mother and baby in person.

## Children's Books

A simple way to introduce breastfeeding to an older baby or toddler is through picture books. These books portray breastfeeding as warm and loving, and the normal way that mothers care for their young. Some children's books show human mothers and babies, some show animals, and others have both. See the Library page on my website for some of my favorites.

## Videos and DVDs

A DVD or online video can take things a step further by portraying breastfeeding in action. It offers both you and your older baby a chance to view latching up close, an opportunity most of us never see until it is our own baby nursing on our breast. Again, check out my website for DVD recommendations and links to online videos.

## Playtime

Playtime with an older baby or toddler can be an opportunity to model breastfeeding with dolls or plush animals. The mother and baby animals don't even have to be the same species—the key is modeling the breastfeeding relationship through play. While specialized dolls or plush animals are not necessary, they are available. For instance, Nursing Nina Cat and Nursing Nana Dog are plush animal mamas and their litters. The kittens or puppies latch onto their mother with magnets.

## Make Bottle-feeding More Like Breastfeeding

The remainder of this chapter is about bridging the gap between bottle-feeding, most likely the way your baby is currently being fed if she is not breastfeeding; and breastfeeding, the way you ultimately wish to feed your baby. If we introduce bottle-feeding techniques that make bottle-feeding more like breastfeeding and breastfeeding techniques that make breastfeeding more like bottle-feeding, we can help your baby to breastfeed by meeting in the middle.

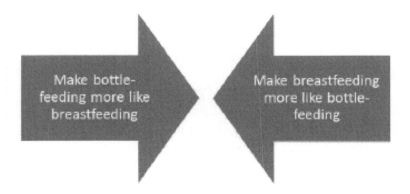

You may have heard the terms "nipple confusion," "nipple preference," or "flow preference." They refer to the difficulty babies can have breastfeeding after being given bottles or pacifiers. Using a bottle or pacifier is a very different experience for the baby than breastfeeding. Often, babies will become frustrated at the breast because they expect it to be like the bottle that they are accustomed to. Dee Kassing, IBCLC (2002) suggests that we can bridge the gap between bottle-feeding and breastfeeding by making bottle-feeding as close to breastfeeding as possible. The Kassing Method is the foundation for the techniques suggested in this chapter.

## Bottle-feed Skin to Skin

Bottle-feeding in a breastfeeding position was introduced in the previous chapter. I recommended bottle-feeding skin to skin, cradling your baby close to you with her cheek on your bare breast. It bears repeating here since it is crucial component in making bottle-feeding more like breastfeeding. Bottle-feeding in such an intimate way also helps to build attachment between you and your new baby.

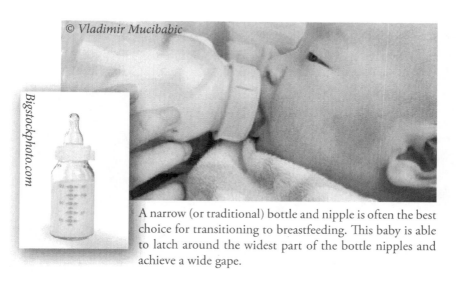

© Vladimir Mucibabic

Bigstockphoto.com

A narrow (or traditional) bottle and nipple is often the best choice for transitioning to breastfeeding. This baby is able to latch around the widest part of the bottle nipples and achieve a wide gape.

## Choose a Bottle Nipple Most Like the Real Thing

Choose a bottle nipple shape that is most like a mother's nipple in the baby's mouth. This type of bottle nipple is not one that looks like mother's breast and nipple, since a mother's areola is very elastic, and so the breast/nipple takes on a very different shape during breastfeeding than the shape that you see. We have observed this on ultrasound videos of breastfeeding babies. Don't be taken in by marketing on the packaging that claims the bottle is "best for breastfeeding." Many of these bottles and nipples are so wide that the baby is only able to take in the tip of the nipple, ending up with a narrow gape. When a baby uses a narrow gape with breastfeeding, she can only take in a small amount of breast tissue, which means she won't get much milk and your nipples may feel really painful. Start with a nipple that gradually widens into a narrow base, approximately 1 inch (25mm) in diameter. The key is to watch how your baby is able to latch onto the nipple: her mouth should be wide with her lips flanged. If baby

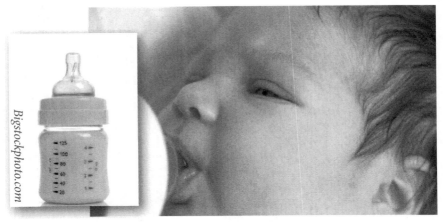

*Bigstockphoto.com*

A wide bottle and nipple may be advertised as most like the breastfeed, but this is often misleading. This baby has a narrow gape on a wide-based bottle, because he is only able to latch onto the narrow tip.

is flattening the bottle nipple, or expressed milk or formula is leaking from the corners of baby's mouth, try a differently shaped bottle nipple (Peterson & Harmer, 2010).

Transition your baby to the newborn or slowest-flow bottle nipple regardless of the age of your baby. Mother's nipples are slow flow and the flow from the breast doesn't change with the age of the baby. There is no standard for what is considered a newborn or slow-flow bottle nipple, so it may be helpful to experiment by filling a bottle with water and checking that the water slowly drips from the bottle nipple.

## Position Baby and Bottle to do the Work of Breastfeeding

Most babies are bottle-fed cradled in a reclined position with the end of the bottle raised so that gravity helps the expressed milk or formula to flow. In breastfeeding, the baby has to do all of the work in extracting the milk from the breast. In order to make bottle-feeding more like breastfeeding, position baby and bottle so that baby's effort, rather than gravity, moves the expressed milk or formula from the bottle into the baby's mouth just as it does when baby is breast-

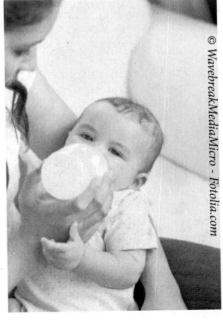

Baby is positioned upright so that her effort, rather than gravity, moves the expressed milk or formula into her mouth.

111

feeding. Baby can be positioned upright on your thigh with your supporting hand cradling the base of her neck and your forearm supporting her back; or the baby can lie prone on her mother's chest and abdomen as her mother is lying back in a semi-reclined position. A narrow, angled bottle may work well when mother is lying back (A. Estorino Uribasterra, personal communication, October 27, 2011). The bottle is positioned so that it is as close to horizontal as possible, tipping just enough so that the level of the expressed milk or formula is even with the baby's lips. It is not necessary to elevate the bottle so that there is no air in the nipple.

**Wait for an Open Mouth**

Wait for baby to open her mouth wide before inserting bottle nipple. Unlike a firm nipple on a bottle, the breast cannot be pushed into a baby's mouth: the baby has to open wide to take in the breast. Rather than pushing the bottle nipple into the baby's mouth, stroke the nipple down the center of the baby's lips to trigger her to open her mouth wide. Then insert the nipple deeply into the baby's mouth so that she takes in both the tip and the wide base of the bottle nipple. If the baby cannot take in the wide base of the nipple, then try a nipple with a base that is narrower.

**Delay the Flow**

When a mother is breastfeeding, the baby must suckle from the breast for a minute or so before her milk starts to flow. Babies who are used to the immediate flow from the bottle may become so frustrated with the lack of immediate flow at the breast that they will not continue to suckle at the breast long enough to for the milk to flow, or let-down. While bottle-feeding, a mother can simulate the wait for mother's milk to let-down by starting the feeding with the bottle tipped down so that no expressed milk or formula enters the nipple. Allow the baby to suckle on the empty nipple for a minute or so before raising the bottle so that expressed milk or formula enters the nipple.

## Switch Sides

Switch sides at least one time during the feeding to accustom baby to feeding on different sides just as with breastfeeding.

## Pace the Feeding

When a baby breastfeeds, the baby lets her mother know when she has had enough. This communication between baby and mother is one of the ways breastfeeding helps develop a trusting relationship between mother and baby. It also sets the foundation for good eating habits! With bottle-feeding, it is tempting for the mother to manage the feeding because she knows how much expressed milk or formula the baby is drinking. Instead, let the baby be in charge of how much expressed milk or formula she drinks. Periodically throughout the feeding, and any time baby indicates distress, either tip the bottle down slightly so that the expressed milk or formula runs out of the nipple back into the bottle, or gently remove the bottle from the baby's mouth, resting the nipple against the baby's lips so she knows the nipple is still there. If the nipple is removed from the baby's mouth, and she does not open her mouth to reinsert the nipple, your baby has indicated that the feeding is over. Your baby may be ready to end a feeding even though there is still expressed milk or formula left in the bottle. If your baby has left expressed milk in the bottle, there is no need to throw that liquid gold away! Just put it in the refrigerator until the next feeding.

Pacing the feeding emulates breastfeeding in another way as well. When a mother breastfeeds, she experiences several let-downs, or milk ejections. Whenever her milk lets down, the flow increases, then slowly decreases until the next let-down. When we pace bottle-feeding, it can also ebb and flow as in breastfeeding.

For most mothers, working with bottle-feeding will help to transition their babies to breastfeeding. Other mothers may benefit from using another feeding device altogether. Sometimes, simply switching to another feeding tool temporarily, such as finger-feeding or cup-feeding, lets the baby know that there is more than one way to get food. (See Chapter 13, Supplementation, for more information on using these feeding tools.) Once the baby realizes that food can come from another source besides the bottle, she may become open to accepting the breast (Newman, 2011).

## Make Breastfeeding More Like Bottle-Feeding

We have discussed how to bridge the gap between bottle-feeding and breastfeeding by making bottle-feeding more like breastfeeding. The gap can also be bridged from the other direction by making breastfeeding more like bottle-feeding.

### Creating a Firm, Protruding Breast

If your baby is bottle-fed, she is used to latching onto a firm and protruding nipple. If your baby is having difficulty latching onto your breast, you can make it easier for your baby to latch by making your own nipple and breast more firm and protruding.

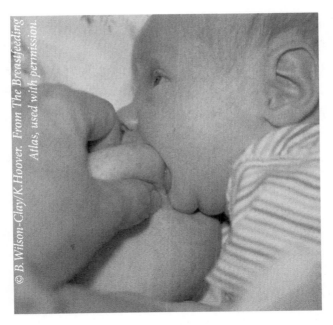

© B.Wilson-Clay/K.Hoover. From The Breastfeeding Atlas, used with permission.

A mother can make a "breast sandwich" so that her nipple is more firm and protruding, and easier for the baby to latch on to.

- **Breast Sandwich.** The breast sandwich is a term developed by Diane Wiessinger, IBCLC, when she observed how people take a bite from a big sandwich: they compress the sandwich and then tip their head back to open their mouths as wide as possible. Diane decided to apply this observation to helping mothers and babies with breastfeeding. She suggests that the mother cup her breast with her thumb aligned with the placement of baby's upper lip and the remaining fingers aligned with the placement of baby's lower lip. The fingers are placed close enough to the nipple to shape it and the surrounding breast tissue, but not so close that they are in the way of the baby's mouth. Then, mother compresses the breast tissue while pulling back slightly towards the chest wall. In this way,

115

she has created a firm, protruding breast for her baby to latch onto. A mother can encourage her baby to tip her head back to achieve the widest open mouth by touching her nipple to the baby's philtrum (the indent between the nose and upper lip) so that baby has to reach up to grasp the nipple.

- **Nipple Shield**. A nipple shield is a thin silicone shield that can be placed over the nipple and areola area. While thin and flexible, it provides a firmer breast for the baby to latch onto and, for babies accustomed to a bottle, a similar feel to the bottle nipple. Some mothers will use the nipple shield as long as their baby is breastfeeding. Most mothers, however, will eventually be able to wean the baby from the nipple shield to breastfeeding from the bare breast. Some babies will wean easily from the nipple shield, while others need a bit of coercing.

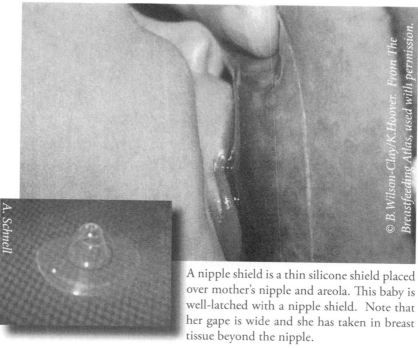

A. Schnell

© B. Wilson-Clay/K.Hoover. From The Breastfeeding Atlas, used with permission.

A nipple shield is a thin silicone shield placed over mother's nipple and areola. This baby is well-latched with a nipple shield. Note that her gape is wide and she has taken in breast tissue beyond the nipple.

*How to use a nipple shield*: Rinse the shield under warm water, if desired, to help the shield stay attached to the breast. Use the inside-out trick developed by Linda Pohl, PE, IBCLC, to help the shield attach and pull mother's nipple into the teat: turn the shield partially inside-out so that the teat is partly inverted and place over mother's nipple; then evert the nipple shield to create a suction, pulling mother's nipple into the teat. Once the nipple shield is in place, position the baby so that her philtrum (the indent between the nose and the upper lip) touches the teat of the nipple shield. This position encourages the baby to tilt her head up to open wide for the nipple (Genna, 2009).

Use of a nipple shield is controversial. Some experts are concerned that a baby will not transfer milk as well with a nipple shield, while others have little concern about milk transfer with the shield. One study on preterm babies even found that the nipple shield helped babies to latch better so that they transferred more milk with the shield than without one (Meier et al., 2000; Powers & Tapia, 2012). In my private practice, I have seen babies drink much more milk with the nipple shield than without. I have also seen babies who were able to latch onto the breast with the nipple shield when they could not latch onto the bare breast, but they were still not able to get any milk from the breast. A nipple shield should be used with caution and under the supervision of a lactation consultant.

## Immediate Reinforcement

Often, a bottle-fed baby learning to breastfeed will latch on, suckle once or twice, and then release the nipple in frustration. This is also very frustrating for the mother who exclaims, "You had it. Why did you let it go?!" The baby may have let it go because she did not get any immediate reinforcement for her efforts. She didn't get any milk because it takes several suckles for mother's milk to let down. Babies who are accustomed to breastfeeding expect this; babies who are accustomed to bottle-feeding expect immediate flow (unless their mother has been delaying the flow when bottle-feeding, as described above). In this case, we can encourage baby to continue suckling by providing immediate flow with breastfeeding.

If you are producing a significant amount of milk, you can hand express before offering the breast in order to start the milk flowing. In addition to the reinforcement of milk flowing immediately upon latching, a few drops of your expressed milk on your nipple can be very enticing to your baby. She is likely to lick those drops off your nipple, and the process of latching is rolling. If you are using a nipple shield, you can hand express into the shield by tipping the teat upward after it has been attached, then hand expressing a little bit of milk into it to entice the baby with an immediate reward for latching (E. O'Reilly, personal communication, June 22, 2010). Some other methods for helping the milk to flow more quickly are to massage your breasts, or to apply a warm, moist washcloth to your breasts just before offering them to the baby.

If you are not producing a significant amount of milk, then you may supplement your milk production by using a feeding tube at the breast, as described below. When a mother supplements with a feeding tube at the breast, she can help the expressed milk or formula to flow from the tubing immediately if that encourages the baby to remain latched, or she can allow the baby to pull the expressed milk or formula through the tubing by suckling for a minute or so as if baby was triggering a let-down. The type of at-breast supplementer the mother uses will determine how she may elicit the expressed milk or formula to reach the end of the tubing before the baby has latched on and suckled long enough to pull it through. One way to draw the expressed milk or formula through any type of at-breast supplementer before baby is suckling is for mother to suck on the tubing herself, if she is comfortable doing so, until the expressed milk or formula reaches the end of the tubing.

## Increase Flow at the Breast

Unlike bottle-feeding, breastfeeding is always slow flow. When milk production is lower than normal (which is usually the case for mothers who induce lactation), the flow of the milk from the breasts is even slower than normal. Your baby may be more interested in breastfeeding if you help the milk to flow more easily.

- **Breast Compression.** Once the baby has latched, you can provide further reinforcement by increasing the flow of milk from your breasts using a technique called breast compression. Breast compression involves gently squeezing the breast while breastfeeding to help push the milk out and to the baby. See Chapter 11, Physical Techniques for Inducing Lactation, for more information on how to use breast compression.

- **Supplementing at the Breast**. We discussed above that babies are more apt to learn to breastfeed when they are not too hungry. However, some babies–especially younger ones– will not be interested in the breast unless they are rewarded with an ample flow of milk. If you are not producing a significant amount of milk, you can supplement what your breasts produce by using a feeding tube at the breast. The feeding tube can be a homemade device or a commercial at-breast supplementer, such as the Lact-Aid or Supplemental Nursing System (SNS). The feeding tube can even be used under a nipple shield. For more information on at-breast supplementers see Chapter 11, Physical Techniques for Inducing Lactation, and Chapter 13, Supplementation.

## Putting It All Together

You and your lactation consultant can work together to find an approach to help your baby to breastfeed. Several breastfeeding experts have found the following sequence successful in transitioning older adopted babies to the breast.

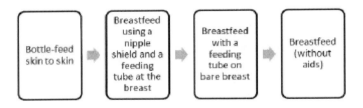

Many mothers have had difficulty getting their babies to latch—whether they have birthed their babies or not. Being willing to keep trying, experiment with various techniques, and get help from an expert will be the keys to your eventual success. Some babies, especially those who start breastfeeding when they are older, may never latch. Yet many babies, after days, weeks, or months of trying, eventually learn to breastfeed. It can be very worth the effort and the wait!

# Section III

# Making Milk—
# Nourishing from the
# Breast

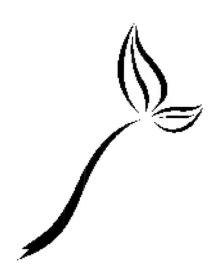

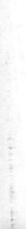

# Chapter 9

# MAKING MILK: WHAT TO EXPECT

Mothering success is not measured in ounces–or drops–of milk that flow from breast to mouth. It's measured in the love that flows between mother and baby (Cassar-Uhl, 2012).

This chapter is devoted to answering some of the questions you may have about what to expect from inducing lactation. Be forewarned: mothers have experienced such a wide range of outcomes when inducing lactation that it is very difficult to predict what any one mother's outcome will be. The one answer I can provide is that a mother who has very specific expectations with regard to milk production when inducing lactation is likely to be disappointed. I encourage you to go into this endeavor with an open mind, believing that any amount of milk you produce will be supremely beneficial to your baby.

## How Much Milk Will I Produce?

Usually the first question expectant mothers ask me about inducing lactation is, "How much milk will I make?" I would love to tell them a certain number of ounces per day, or a percentage of their baby's intake. I can only provide a broad range: most mothers from

Western countries who induce lactation produce 25% to 75% of their baby's nutritional needs (Avery, 2012[1]; Hormann, 1977). Some mothers—and I know of a few, me included—have been able to provide 100% of their baby's nutritional needs. Some mothers are not able to produce any milk.

Why such a broad range of outcomes for mothers inducing lactation? Milk production is influenced by many factors, some of which you may have control over, and some that you do not.

- Mother's motivation
- Mother's previous breastfeeding experience
- Breastfeeding support
- Mother's health
- Condition of mother's breasts
- Parenting practices
- Frequency and effectiveness of nipple stimulation and milk removal
- Use of galactogogues (herbs or medications that may enhance milk production)

## Mother's Motivation

Motivation is perhaps the most important determinant of the amount of milk a mother will produce by inducing lactation. When breastfeeding is really important to a mother, her body is much more likely to respond to her efforts, even when other important factors for milk production are lacking (El-Taweel, 2012; WHO, 1998).

## Anat's Story: Highly Motivated to Breastfeed an Ill Baby

*Anat, a mother by birth to several older children, became a foster*

[1] Posthumous reference to her website

*mother to baby Kamila when Kamila's birthmother died in childbirth. Kamila was a very ill baby, suffering from hydrocephalus (water on the brain) and experiencing frequent, severe convulsions as a result. Anat was very nurturing, sensitive, and responsive to Kamila's special needs. Despite her desires, Anat's husband was opposed to Anat breastfeeding Kamila. However, Anat had a secret. During the middle of the night, while preparing Kamila's bottle of formula, Anat would latch Kamila at the breast to soothe her while she waited for her bottle. After just a few weeks of putting Kamila to the breast just once per day, Anat began producing milk. With just one nursing session per day, Kamila's convulsions became much less frequent and less severe.*

## Mother's Prior Breastfeeding Experience

Mothers who have breastfed prior babies tend to produce more milk (Auerbach, 1981). This statement is even true for mothers who have given birth to their nursling because each time a mother is pregnant and/or breastfeeds, she builds glandular breast tissue. The shorter the amount of time since a mother last breastfed, the more milk a mother is likely to produce (WHO, 1998). In addition to the physiological advantage, a mother with previous breastfeeding experience has confidence in her ability to breastfeed. She has knowledge and resources accrued from her previous breastfeeding experiences that provide a foundation for breastfeeding success.

## Breastfeeding Culture

Research has shown that mothers from developing countries, where breastfeeding is often the cultural norm, produce more milk. These mothers have the support of their entire community. They are confident in their ability to breastfeed, because they grew up in an environment where breastfeeding was just a normal part of life. They saw their mothers, sisters, aunts, cousins, and friends all publicly breastfeeding as part of the daily routine of caring for a baby. Mothers from these countries are more likely to parent in ways that support breastfeeding. They are also less likely to have alternatives, such as bottles and infant formula, readily available. Despite the lack of availability of breast pumps and medications to enhance milk production, these mothers still tend to make more milk than mothers in developed countries (Gribble, 2004).

If you don't live in a breastfeeding culture—and many of you reading this book don't—you can still achieve the degree of milk production that the mothers in developing countries do by participating within a breastfeeding culture-within-a-culture. This usually happens within the context of a close extended family of breastfeeding mothers, or a breastfeeding mothers' group, such as La Leche League (Thorley, 2004). See Chapter 2, A Community of Support, for more information.

**Mother's Health**

In general, a mother who is healthy will produce more milk. Some key ingredients for generous milk production are:

- **Rest.** If your baby hasn't arrived yet, bank as many hours of sleep as you can. These will become precious later. If your baby has arrived, sleep when your baby sleeps. Get help around the house if possible to free up your time to rest when your baby doesn't need you.
- **Relaxation.** Easier said than done as you are expecting your

baby's arrival, or if you have a new baby! If you are feeling stressed, breathe deeply for several minutes and imagine yourself in a calm place such as the beach, your favorite cozy chair, or wherever you feel most relaxed. Exercise. Spend time with friends. Although you won't have as much time as before baby, don't give up your hobbies and interests.

- **Diet.** Over 50 years ago, La Leche League began advising mothers, "Good nutrition means eating a well-balanced and varied diet of foods in as close to their natural state as possible" (LLL, 2006). These are excellent dietary guidelines for breastfeeding mothers—and for everyone else as well. If you would like to take diet a step further, foods with particular reputations for increasing milk production are described in Chapter 12, Medications for Inducing Lactation.

- **Thirst.** Drink healthy beverages, such as water, herbal teas[2], and juices. Drink to thirst, but not past it. It is a common misconception that the more a mother drinks, the more milk she will make.

Your health history can provide clues regarding your ability to produce milk. If you are a woman who is infertile due to hormonal issues, these same issues can affect your ability to make milk. Some common causes of infertility that can affect milk production are Polycystic Ovarian Syndrome (PCOS), luteal phase defect (LPD), pituitary issues, thyroid dysfunction, diabetes, and age. If you have any of these health issues, seek the support of your healthcare practitioner. Make sure your medications are doing their jobs. Alternative healthcare practitioners, such as chiropractors, acupuncturists, natu-

---

[2] Although herbal teas are generally compatible with breastfeeding, avoid peppermint or spearmint teas as mint can actually suppress milk production.

ropaths, homeopaths, herbalists, and doctors of Chinese Medicine, can also be helpful in supporting balanced hormones and overall health. For more information regarding hormonal issues and milk production, see *The Breastfeeding Mother's Guide to Making More Milk* (West & Marasco, 2009).

## The Condition of Mother's Breasts

Certain conditions can limit the ability of your breasts to make milk.

- **A History of Breast Surgery.** Breast surgery can sever or damage milk ducts, and the nerves in and around the breasts. It may also result in a decreased amount of glandular breast tissue.
- **A History of Breast Injury.** Breast injury may result in damage to the milk ducts or nerves in the breasts.
- **Hypoplasia/Insufficient Glandular Tissue.** Some mothers have a condition called breast hypoplasia, also known as insufficient glandular tissue (IGT), in which their glandular breast tissue has not fully developed. If your breasts have an unusual shape or large spacing between them, your lactation consultant can examine your breasts for signs of hypoplasia/IGT.

## Parenting Practices

Does it seem surprising that how you parent can influence a physiological process like lactation? Using any of the parenting tools for latching and attaching introduced in Chapter 6, such as babywearing, co-sleeping, or co-bathing, boosts levels of oxytocin, an essential hormone for lactation, since oxytocin increases whenever mother and baby are in close body contact. Furthermore, using any of these tools often leads to more frequent breastfeeding, a key to good milk production.

## Frequency and Effectiveness of Breast Stimulation and Milk Removal

The primary and most effective type of breast stimulation and milk removal is a baby who is breastfeeding often and breastfeeding well. For mothers who are supplementing breastfeeding with expressed milk or formula, the use of an at-breast supplementer (versus a bottle or other supplemental feeding method) can increase both the quality and quantity of suckling from the breast (Genna, 2009). More information regarding at-breast supplementers is provided in Chapter 13, Supplementation.

Breast stimulation and milk removal can also happen using a breast pump, with hand expression, or by partner suckling. Often, mothers will use these techniques prior to baby's arrival to initiate lactation, as well as after baby arrives to further increase milk production. For mothers inducing lactation prior to baby's arrival, the amount of milk produced by pumping or hand expressing does not necessarily indicate the amount of milk a mother will be able to produce once she is breastfeeding (Starr, 2008). Chapter 11, Physical Techniques for Inducing Lactation, describes each of these milk-making techniques in detail.

### Use of Galactogogues

Galactogogues can be herbal or pharmaceutical medications, or foods reputed to increase milk production. Taking galactogogues may increase your milk production, and the pharmaceutical medication Domperidone has been shown to be the most effective of the galactogogues. If you have run the gamut of fertility treatments, you may find the idea of using medications to induce lactation is nothing compared to the heavy-duty hormones that you took during fertility treatments, or you may feel that you are through with taking medications. See Chapter 12, Medications for Inducing Lactation, for more

**For Mothers Using Hormonal Medications Prior to Inducing Lactation**

*Birth Control*

If a mother is fertile, she may need to reconsider her birth control method while inducing lactation. Hormonal birth control in the form of a birth control pill, sub-dermal implant, patch, vaginal ring, or hormonal intrauterine device (IUD) inflates progesterone and, in some cases, estrogen levels. Increased levels of progesterone and estrogen suppress milk production. While estrogen-containing hormonal birth control is never recommended for breastfeeding mothers, some progesterone-only birth control methods are considered acceptable while breastfeeding if baby is older than six weeks old.[3] However, some mothers have reported that their milk production decreased with the use of progestin-only birth control (Hale, 2012; West & Marasco, 2009). As a result, progestin-only birth control is not recommended for moth-

[3] Progestin-only birth control poses health concerns for the development in babies younger than six weeks due to the small amount of the hormone that passes into the milk. (WHO, Department of Reproductive Health and Research, 2008)

ers, such as those inducing lactation, who wish to increase their milk production. Some recommended birth control methods for breastfeeding mothers are Natural Family Planning; barrier methods (condoms, diaphragms, contraceptive sponges, and cervical caps) and spermicides; non-hormonal IUDs; or surgical sterilization (vasectomy and tubal ligation) (Mohrbacher, 2010).

Now here's the confusing part: although hormonal birth control methods, including the birth control pill, are not recommended for mothers who are lactating, a birth control pill can be used to help build breast tissue prior to initiating lactation. More information on the use of a birth control pill for this purpose will be discussed in Chapter 12, Medications for Inducing Lactation.

### Hormone Replacement Therapy

A woman who is post-menopausal can still produce milk. Reproductive organs are not necessary to make milk--all that is needed is a functioning pituitary gland. A woman on hormone replacement therapy may decide to adjust her medications when inducing lactation. The birth control pill, if that is part of the plan to induce lactation, may alleviate menopausal symptoms and eliminate the need for hormone replacement therapy. If you have menopausal symptoms while inducing lactation, consuming soy products may help. Eat only enough soy products to eliminate your symptoms—too much soy can decrease milk production (Goldfarb & Newman, accessed October 31, 2012).

**Samantha's Story:  Lactation Suppressed by Hormonal Contraceptive**

*When Samantha came to see me, she had already educated herself on how to induce lactation.  Although she had already breastfed several biological children, and had been pumping regularly for over a month, she did not observe any changes in her breasts in preparation for lactation. She was using a vaginal ring contraceptive.*

information on using galactogogues.

## How Long Will It Take?

In most cases, it takes at least a month to prepare the breasts before they can make milk.  Occasionally, it can take longer.  Once the breasts begin making milk, as breast stimulation and milk removal continue, the amount of milk produced will increase from droplets to sprays of milk.  The amount of time it takes to start producing the first droplets of milk does not indicate the amount of milk you will be able to eventually produce (Starr, 2008).  In one case report, an adoptive mother began inducing lactation when her baby was 10 days old.  No noticeable milk was produced until the baby was four months old.  Within a week, the mother was making enough milk to exclusively breastfeed her baby (Cheales-Siebenaler, 1999).

## Is the Composition of the Milk Different When a Mother Induces Lactation?

Human milk contains over 200 components especially designed to meet the needs of infants.  Only one study, including only two mothers who induced lactation, has investigated the composition of milk in mothers who have induced lactation. The two mothers in the study produced milk similar in composition to that of mothers who birthed their babies (Kulski et al., 1981).

Although most mothers who induce lactation do not reach full milk production, their milk contains the same number of antibodies and other immune factors as that of mothers who birth and exclusively breastfeed their babies because human milk always provides full immunities, regardless of level of milk production (Wiessinger et al., 2010).

### Initial Secretions

In a study of 240 mothers who induced lactation, researchers found that the initial secretions from the breast varied among mothers from clear, to colostrum-like (thick and yellow), to milky. Women who had lactated for previous babies were more likely to produce milky secretions, whereas women who had not lactated before were more likely to produce clear or colostrum-like secretions. Most mothers will initially express milk that is clear and watery, and then becomes more opaque over time (Auerbach, 1981). The composition of the first droplets of milk is not significant, however, because it is not generally enough to collect.

## How Will Inducing Lactation Affect My Body and My Emotions?

As your milk production begins and then increases, you may notice changes in your body and your emotions as you adjust hormonally and physiologically to breastfeeding. These changes are a good thing: they mean your body is shifting into milk-making mode!

## Menstrual Changes

As your hormones adjust for lactation, your periods may stop or become irregular. Breastfeeding, especially in the first months, usually prevents menstruation in mothers who have given birth. For mothers who are inducing lactation, anything goes. Some mothers will experience no periods while breastfeeding; others will experience shorter, lighter, or missed periods; while others will not experience any interruption in their cycles (Amica & Finley, 1986). Some mothers who have induced lactation (as well as mothers who have birthed) will notice a drop or plateau in milk production the few days before menstruation (Avery, 2012[4]). If you are one of these mothers, Pat Gima, IBCLC, suggests taking 500 to 1000 mg of calcium/magnesium per day from ovulation (mid-cycle) to three days into menstruation (West & Marasco, 2009).

## Breast Changes

As you build milk ducts and glandular breast tissue, you may experience changes in how your breasts feel. You may notice breast changes, such as heaviness, enlargement, tenderness, or darkening of the areola.

## Mood Changes

Along with hormonal changes may come mood changes. Often, the breastfeeding hormones prolactin and oxytocin give mother's mood a boost and help decrease stress levels. Sometimes, though, the hormonal changes with lactation (or from the medications used to induce lactation) can leave a mother feeling exhausted, stressed, depressed, or overwhelmed. This is another reason to have a strong support system in place (see Chapters 2 and 3), and to take extra care of yourself during this time (Mohrbacher, 2010).

As you enter the journey of inducing lactation, be ready for your experience to be unique. From the information in this chapter, you may have some idea what to expect, but even more importantly, you will be open to however your experience unfolds. Using the techniques in the following chapters, you have an excellent chance of producing some milk for your special baby.

# Chapter 10

# APPROACHES TO INDUCING LACTATION

Approaches to inducing lactation can be broken down into three steps for making milk without pregnancy and birth. **Steps 1 and 2 are optional**, so the process of inducing lactation can be quite simple or more involved, depending upon your individual values and circumstances.

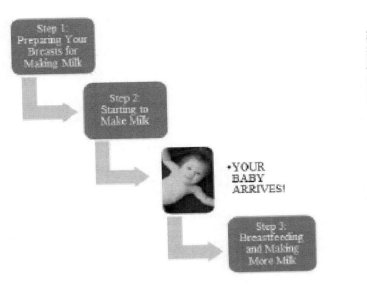

## Step 1: Preparing Your Breasts for Making Milk

You can prepare your breasts for making milk as would occur during a pregnancy. During pregnancy, the milk ducts and glandular tissue in a woman's breasts develop in preparation for breastfeeding. These breast changes result from pregnancy hormones: primarily estrogen, progesterone, and prolactin. A woman who is pregnant will observe these changes in her breasts as enlargement, tenderness, feeling of fullness or increased weight, a darkening of the areola, or an increased elasticity of the nipples (nipples will draw out more easily). These same breast changes can be induced in a mother who is not pregnant. You can artificially boost your hormone levels with pharmaceutical or herbal medications to emulate the hormonal state of pregnancy, or you can physically stimulate your breasts using hand expression, breast massage, nipple manipulation, or partner stimulation to induce them to develop in preparation for lactation.

## Step 2: Starting to Make Milk Before Your Baby Arrives

This is the exciting point at which you may start producing milk by pumping or hand expressing on a regular basis throughout the day. Taking medications in addition to pumping or hand expressing may increase the amount of milk you produce, but this is always optional. The recommended length of time in Step 2 is about six weeks before baby arrives. Four to six weeks is generally enough time to bring in some milk (Avery, 2012[1]). Planning for six weeks leaves an extra cushion for babies who arrive early. Because Step 2 involves regular (at least eight times per day) pumping or hand expression, spending much more time in this step can be draining. The tricky part is that adoptive and foster mothers don't always have four to six weeks before

[1] Posthumous reference to her website

138

baby arrives. (Other breastfeeding-without-birthing mothers usually do.) Sometimes, a baby arrives much later than expected, and weeks of pumping can turn into months. In other cases, babies can arrive on very short notice. Most birthmothers make their adoption plan in their third trimester, and many don't make an adoption plan until the baby has been born. Many mothers may plan to spend four to six weeks in Step 2, and end up spending considerably less time or no time at all in Step 2. No problem! Putting that beautiful baby to the breast in Step 3 is better than any ol' breast pump any day!

## Step 3: Breastfeeding and Making More Milk

Step 3 begins when your baby has arrived and you begin breastfeeding. A baby who is nursing well is the most effective means for increasing milk production. In order to nurse well, most babies require an ample flow of milk either directly from mother's breasts, or with the help of an at-breast supplementer if mother isn't producing much, or any, milk. An at-breast supplementer typically consists of a tiny feeding tube carrying milk or formula to the nipple from a bag or bottle that hangs around mother's neck. (See Chapter 13, Supplementation, for detailed information on using an at-breast supplementer.) Some mothers will continue to pump following breastfeeding to further stimulate milk production, while other mothers find breastfeeding, pumping, and caring for a new baby to be too much.

As with any of the steps, medications may be helpful, but they are not necessary. If you chose to use medications in Step 2, these will likely be the same ones you will use in Step 3, since the choice of medications is not dependent upon whether the breast pump, mother's hands, or the baby are stimulating the breasts and removing milk.

At this point, if you find you are able to make enough milk for your baby, congratulations! It will still be important to monitor your baby since her nutritional needs will increase as she grows. However, most mothers who induce lactation will need to supplement breast-feeding from the start. Many approaches to inducing lactation call for supplementation with an at-breast supplementer, while others don't specify. (See Chapter 13, Supplementation, for more information about this and other methods of supplementing.)

Breastfeeding experts have suggested several approaches to inducing lactation, often called protocols, based on some or all of these steps. You may find one of the protocols suits you well, or you may choose to create your own. approach by drawing ideas from several of the protocols. While none of the protocols were developed from randomized clinical trials, each is based on the professional recommendations of medical doctors, lactation consultants, and/or research scientists. Each of the protocols has been shaped by the testimonies of the mothers who have used them. Protocols are described below approximately in order of intricacy. Remember, Steps 1 and 2 are always optional.

### The Decision to Start to Induce Lactation after Your Baby Arrives

Most mothers, if they have the choice, will choose to begin inducing lactation before baby arrives. In the context of the protocols, inducing lactation before your baby arrives means including Step 1 or Step 2, or both, in addition to Step 3. This offers many advantages.

- **You may already be making milk when your baby**

**arrives.** Inducing lactation before your baby arrives is very appealing because you will most likely already be producing milk when you meet your baby. If she is arriving as a newborn, even a partial milk supply may be sufficient to meet her needs in the early days. Even if you are not making milk by the time your baby arrives, your breasts have started to prepare for lactation, which can lead to your milk coming in sooner than if you had waited until your baby's arrival to begin inducing lactation.

- **Your stored milk can be used to supplement breastfeeding.** Because most mothers who induce lactation produce a partial milk supply, you will most likely need to supplement breastfeeding. The ideal supplement is your own expressed milk (WHO, 2003). By inducing lactation before your baby's arrival, you can bank your own milk for future use.

- **Inducing lactation before your baby is born is a way to care for her in utero**. When your baby is being cared for in utero by another mother, inducing lactation is one thing that you can do during that time to care for your baby's health and well-being. It is your "pregnancy."

- **Inducing lactation is an opportunity for you to become familiar with your breasts and confident in their ability to make milk**. If you have never breastfed before, inducing lactation prior to your baby's arrival can give you a jump start with feeling comfortable and confident in the ability of your breasts to make milk. What can be a better boost than holding a bottle containing your own milk?

- **You have more time before baby arrives**. Caring for a new baby can be very time consuming! Most mothers have more time to devote to building their milk production before their baby arrives.

### Shelby's Story: Time to Pump

*Shelby was so busy getting ready for the arrival of baby Landon via surrogacy, along with caring for her two older children, that she found little time for pumping. She decided to pump three to four times per day even though at least eight times is recommended for mothers inducing lactation. When baby Landon arrived, Shelby was producing about six ounces per day, a substantial amount but considerably less than baby Landon required. Shelby realized that if she had pumped more often before Landon was born, she might have been able to provide most or all of Landon's nutritional needs with breastfeeding. Instead, she now had even less time than before to work on building her milk production. "Oh, how I wish I listened to you when you told me to pump eight times a day!" Shelby told me.*

Inducing lactation after your baby arrives means skipping Steps 1 and 2 and starting your protocol at Step 3. Although the list of reasons to begin lactation after baby arrives is much shorter than the list of reasons to start before, these few reasons can be pretty significant. Consider your personal circumstances.

- **Plans can fall through**. In the case of surrogacy, plans are generally pretty secure. With adoption, plans may or may not be secure. Your adoption professional can help you evaluate the chances that your plans may fall through. If a mother induces lactation before her baby arrives, she has her milk production and all the hormones associated with that, on top of her incredible loss.

- **Little to no lead time before baby's arrival**. Often with adoption, mothers receive just a day or a few days' notice before it is time to meet their baby. If this is the case for you, your options for inducing lactation ahead of time depend on the protocol you have chosen.

  - The Traditional Protocol does not call for inducing lactation prior to your baby's arrival.

  - If you have chosen the Newman-Goldfarb Protocol, you can begin preparing your breasts for lactation (Step 1) before you know when your baby will arrive. Then, if there is little or no lead time, you can skip (or shorten) the pumping step (Step 2), and go straight to breastfeeding (Step 3) as soon as your baby arrives.

  - If you have chosen a protocol that is not the Traditional Protocol or the Newman-Goldfarb Protocol, you have two options. You can wait for a match with a baby before beginning to induce lactation, and risk not having any time to begin inducing lactation before baby arrives; or you can begin your chosen protocol before getting a match and risk spending many months pumping and/or hand expressing regularly throughout the day. To add some perspective, some mothers by birth exclusively pump: they express their milk with a breast pump six to eight times per day—some mothers for as long as a year--and exclusively bottle-feed their babies their expressed milk.

- **Support arrives after baby arrives**. For working mothers, the law requires that employers provide adequate time and space for mothers to express their milk (usually with a breast pump) throughout the workday. Your employer may be hesitant to provide this type of support if your baby hasn't yet arrived (D. Kassing, personal communication, November 5, 2012). Additionally, if your close family includes experienced breastfeeding mothers, you may feel more comfortable beginning lactation once your baby has arrived and you are surrounded by family support.

## Tamara's Story: A Terrible Loss

*Tamara began inducing lactation when she was matched with a birthmother in Minnesota. She was pumping and taking herbs, and had started producing small quantities of milk when the birthmother abruptly broke contact with the adoption agency. For a few weeks, the agency could not find the birthmother, and the adoption status was up in the air. Tamara contacted me for some guidance: should she continue inducing lactation or not? She decided to continue pumping and taking herbs, but she pumped less frequently. She did not want to close the milk-making factory completely, but it was so emotionally painful to pump milk for a baby that might never come. In the end, Tamara and her husband flew to Minnesota for the birth, they cared for the baby for two days, and then the birthmother decided to keep the baby. This was an unusual, yet terribly heartbreaking situation. When Tamara adopted baby William about a year later, she chose not to induce lactation prior to his arrival.*

## Sandy's Story: A Long Wait

*Sandy and her husband decided to adopt a baby from Vietnam. She induced lactation with great success, producing up to 25 ounces of milk per day! Unfortunately, U.S. Immigration began having difficulties with the Vietnamese agency and closed down adoptions with it. Sandy made a change of plans, and began seeking to adopt in Colombia. Their promised placement date came and went. When this story was documented, it had been six months since Sandy had begun pumping, and still no placement. She had decreased the number of times she was pumping per day, and was able to maintain milk production of 18 ounces per day. "On some days, every time I pump makes me realize that I don't yet have a baby. On other days, I feel that at least it's keeping me connected to the process"* (Behrmann, 2005, p. 59).

The decision whether to induce lactation prior to baby's arrival is not an all-or-nothing choice. As in the stories above,

145

a mother may choose to start to induce lactation based on one of the protocols, but decrease the frequency of the physical techniques and/or increase the length of time in Step 1, Step 2, or both. If you are not following any of the protocols as directed, please consult with your International Board Certified Lactation Consultant (IBCLC) for guidance.

## The Traditional Protocol

The Traditional Protocol for inducing lactation is to breastfeed, breastfeed, breastfeed. Induced lactation happens most commonly, most simply, and most successfully in traditional cultures where breastfeeding is the cultural norm and breast pumps, at-breast supplementers, bottles, and medications are not likely to be readily available. In these cultures, mothers simply breastfeed very frequently (10 to 14 times per day—even more in some cases), and supplement with cup- or spoon-feeding as needed. It is common in traditional cultures for adoptive mothers (who are typically mothers who have breastfed previous babies by birth) to produce a full milk supply.

| | Start Time Before Baby's Expected Arrival | Physical Techniques | Medications |
|---|---|---|---|
| Step 1: Preparing your breast for making milk | N/A | -none- | -none- |

| Step 2: Starting to make milk before baby arrives | N/A | -none- | -none- |
|---|---|---|---|
| Step 3: Breastfeeding and making more milk | When baby arrives | Breastfeed<br>Breast massage (in some cultures) | |

(Abejide et al., 1997)

# The Avery Protocol

The Avery Protocol is based on the recommendations of Jimmie Lynn Avery, adoptive mother and developer of the Lact-Aid at-breast supplementer. Avery, together with Kathleen Auerbach, conducted a survey of 240 adoptive mothers who had induced lactation. Avery and Auerbach found that approximately two thirds of the mothers in their survey estimated that they were producing 50% to 75% of their baby's nutrition after 10 to 12 weeks of nursing. Like the Traditional Protocol, the Avery Protocol is rather simple in that it doesn't go through all three steps, and requires no medications of any kind. Avery emphasizes the importance of using the time before baby arrives to become "emotionally attuned to the giving, touching, intimacy of nursing." Her recommendations emphasize manual stimulation of the breasts, as well as the valuable role of the partner in breast and nipple stimulation.

| | Start Time Before Baby's Expected Arrival | Physical Techniques | Medications |
|---|---|---|---|
| **Step 1: Preparing your breast for making milk** | N/A | -none- | -none- |
| **Step 2: Starting to make milk before baby arrives** | At least one month | Hand expression<br><br>Breast massage<br><br>Nipple manipulation<br><br>Partner stimulation | -none- |
| **Step 3: Breastfeeding and making more milk** | When baby arrives | Breastfeed with an at-breast supplementer | |

(Avery, 2012; Auerbach & Avery, 1981)

# The Pumping Protocol

The Pumping Protocol, like the previous protocols, requires only physical techniques--no medications--to induce lactation. I consider it more advanced than the previous protocols because it calls for the use of an electric breast pump.

| | Start Time Before Baby's Expected Arrival | Physical Techniques | Medications |
|---|---|---|---|
| **Step 1: Preparing your breast for making milk** | 8-10 weeks | Breast massage<br>Nipple manipulation | -none- |

| Step 2: Starting to make milk before baby arrives | 6 weeks | Pump | -none- |
|---|---|---|---|
| Step 3: Breastfeeding and making more milk | When baby arrives | Breastfeed with an at-breast supplementer<br><br>Pump (as needed and desired) | |

(West & Marasco, 2009)

# The Herbal Protocol

The Herbal Protocol, as the name suggests, calls for herbs that support milk production–a good option for many mothers who have chosen to use herbal medications, but not pharmaceuticals, for inducing lactation. Herbs that support milk production, known as herbal galactogogues, are reputed to build breast tissue, increase milk production, or assist milk ejection (let-down). (See Chapter 12, Medications for Inducing Lactation, and Appendix C, Potential Side Effects and Safety Cautions for Herbal Galactogogues, for more information.)

While goat's rue is recommended for building breast tissue in Step 1, most mothers find a combination of herbs most helpful once they are physically stimulating the breasts to make milk in steps 2 and 3. Lisa Marasco, MS, IBCLC, recommends the following quality herbal combinations for mothers who are inducing lactation: More Milk Special Blend by Motherlove Herbals, Adoptive Milk in Formula by Simply Herbal, or Mother's Lactaflow by Wise Woman Herbals (2012)[1].

149

Another option is to create your own herbal combination including alfalfa, blessed thistle, fennel, fenugreek, goat's rue, saw palmetto, and/or shatavari. Andrea, an adoptive mother with an abundant milk supply, explained to me that she developed her own combination of herbs by trying various herbs and choosing only those that "felt like what my body needed."

| | Start Time Before Baby's Expected Arrival | Physical Techniques | Medications |
|---|---|---|---|
| **Step 1: Preparing your breast for making milk** | 2 to 3 months | -none- | Goat's Rue |
| **Step 2: Starting to make milk before baby arrives** | 1 to 2 months (after 1 month in Step 1) | Pump Hand expression Nipple manipulation | A quality combination of herbal galactogogues |
| **Step 3: Breastfeeding and making more milk** | When baby arrives | Breastfeed | |

(S. Cox, Motherlove Herbals, personal communication, July 22, 2011 and November 28, 2012)

---

[1] More Milk Special Blend contains goat's rue, fenugreek, blessed thistle, nettle, and fennel. Adoptive Milk in Formula contains goat's rue, alfalfa, blessed thistle, borage, lactuca virosa, shatavari, fenugreek, and saw palmetto. Mother's Lactaflow contains fennel, fenugreek, blessed thistle, and goat's rue. All are herbal tinctures.

# The Newman-Goldfarb Protocols

The Newman-Goldfarb Protocols for Induced Lactation© are the most intricate of the established protocols: steps include the use of a multi-user breast pump, herbal or pharmaceutical medications, and an at-breast supplementer. Regardless of how long a mother has until her baby arrives, she can start these protocols right away. These protocols for inducing lactation are very popular in Western countries due to their effectiveness: most mothers using the Newman-Goldfarb Protocol for at least 3.5 months will produce 60% to 100% of their babies' nutritional needs (Mohrbacher, 2010).

|  | Start Time Before Baby's Expected Arrival | Physical Techniques | Medications |
|---|---|---|---|
| **Step 1: Preparing your breast for making milk** | 3.5 months or more | -none- | BCP -or- Progesterone -or- Progesterone and Goat's rue  Domperidone |
| **Step 2: Starting to make milk before baby arrives** | 6 to 8 weeks | Pump *with breast massage*  Partner timulation | Domperidone -or- Fenugreek and Blessed Thistle |
| **Step 3: Breastfeeding and making more milk** | When baby arrives | Breastfeed with breast compression and/ or an at-breast supplementer |  |

(Newman & Goldfarb, accessed October 26, 2012; Newman, MD, personal communication, December 15, 2012)

# Creating Your Own Protocol

You may find that one of the above protocols fits the bill. If not, together with your International Board Certified Lactation Consultant (IBCLC), you can create a protocol that suits your individual situation and values. I suggest that you use the other protocols as a guide.

| | Start Time Before Baby's Expected Arrival | Physical Techniques | Medications |
|---|---|---|---|
| **Step 1: Preparing your breast for making milk** | Any time before baby arrives | ☐ Hand expression<br>☐ Breast massage<br>☐ Nipple manipulation<br>☐ Partner stimulation<br>☐ None of the above | ☐ Birth control pill -or- progesterone -or- progesterone and goat's rue -or- goat's rue<br>☐ Domperidone<br>☐ None of the above |
| **Step 2: Starting to make milk before baby arrives** | Up to six weeks | ☐ Pump<br>☐ Hand expression<br>☐ None of the above | ☐ Domperidone<br>☐ Alfalfa<br>☐ Blessed Thistle<br>☐ Fennel<br>☐ Fenugreek<br>☐ Goat's rue<br>☐ Saw Palmetto<br>☐ Shatavari<br>☐ None of the above |
| **Step 3: Breastfeeding and making more milk** | When baby arrives | ☑ Breastfeed -or- breastfeed with at-breast supplementer<br>☐ Pump<br>☐ Hand expression | ☐ Domperidone<br>☐ Alfalfa<br>☐ Blessed Thistle<br>☐ Fennel<br>☐ Fenugreek<br>☐ Goat's rue<br>☐ Saw Palmetto<br>☐ Shatavari<br>☐ None of the above |

# Chapter 11

# PHYSICAL TECHNIQUES FOR INDUCING LACTATION

## Breast Stimulation and Milk Removal

The primary, and only necessary techniques for inducing lactation, are frequent and effective breast stimulation and milk removal. That is why the protocols listed in the previous chapter all included physical techniques, while not all called for medications. Physical techniques that can be used to induce lactation include the following.

- Breastfeeding
- Pumping
- Hand expression
- Breast massage
- Nipple manipulation
- Partner stimulation

None of the protocols for inducing lactation introduced in the previous chapter calls for the use of all of these techniques. In fact, breastfeeding is the only physical technique recommended in all of the protocols. For the physical techniques that are part of your chosen protocol (or the individualized protocol you have developed with your lactation consultant), this chapter provides you with detailed information on how to use each one when inducing lactation.

# Breastfeeding

A baby who is breastfeeding well is the most effective way to stimulate a mother's breasts to make milk, or make more milk. It is the stimulus to make milk that a mother's body is designed to respond to. Breastfeeding is the perfect combination of compression and suction, moving in the perfect rhythm. Because babies often don't suckle effectively without an adequate flow of milk, breast compression and/ or using an at-breast supplementer encourage a baby to nurse well when mother doesn't have much milk. If you are having difficulty getting your baby to breastfeed, refer back to Chapters 4 through 8.

## Breast Storage Capacity

The amount of glandular breast tissue that a mother has determines how much milk her breasts can hold at one time, known as "breast storage capacity." All breastfeeding mothers have a breast storage capacity, some larger or smaller than others. Research based on mothers who gave birth has shown that babies of mothers with larger breast storage capacity can fill their tummies on fewer feedings each day, and mothers with smaller breast storage capacity need to feed their babies more frequently to meet their babies' needs. Despite the differences in frequency of feedings, most mothers by birth, whether they have larger or smaller breast storage capacities, can meet their babies' nutritional needs (Mohrbacher & Kendall-Tackett, 2010).

But what about mothers who have not given birth? We know that mothers who induce lactation generally build less glandular breast tissue than mothers who have built glandular breast tissue during pregnancy. Less glandular breast tissue means an extra small storage capacity, and extra small storage capacity means extra-frequent feedings—or more supplementation. We can do the math. Let's say a mother who induces lactation has a breast storage capacity of one ounce per breast. If she breastfeeds (from both breasts) a typical eight times per day, she is providing her baby with about 16 ounces of breastmilk per day. She will need to feed her baby at least nine ounces per day of supplemental milk or formula. What if she breastfeeds 13 times per day? She may not need to supplement at all. This is a tradeoff each mother must make: the time and effort of preparing and feeding a supplement versus the time and effort of breastfeeding more frequently.

## Breastfeeding with Breast Compression

With breast compression, mother gently squeezes her breast as she is nursing to increase the flow of milk to her baby and to help fully empty her breasts. The milk flows more slowly when a mother is producing less milk, so breast compression can be used to temporarily boost the flow of milk. A faster flow of milk encourages baby to suckle longer and more effectively, which helps him get the most milk possible from the breast—and empty breasts further signal the brain to make more milk.

To do breast compression, watch your baby for active suckling and swallowing. When baby is no longer actively suckling/swallowing, gently compress your breast with your thumb wrapped around one side of your breast and the rest of your fingers around the opposite side. Release the compression when the baby is no longer actively suckling and swallowing. Repeat breast compressions as needed (rotating your hand to compress different areas of the breast if desired), until your baby is no longer actively suckling, even with the help of breast compressions (Newman, 2009). See the Links page of my website to link to Dr. Newman's online videos demonstrating breast compression and what active suckling and swallowing—"good drinking"—looks like.

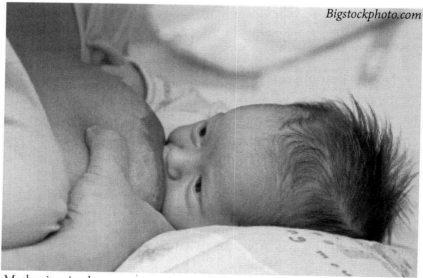

*Bigstockphoto.com*

Mother is using breast compression to increase the flow of milk from the breast.

## Breastfeeding with an At-Breast Supplementer

When a baby is not getting as much milk as he needs from the breast, an at-breast supplementer can act as an external milk duct, allowing baby to continue receiving nourishment and nurturing at mother's breast while supplementing her milk supply with additional expressed milk or formula. Supplementing at the breast stimulates the breasts to make more milk in several ways: baby is at the breast for a longer period of time, baby is providing more breast stimulation by suckling more actively and effectively when encouraged by an ample flow of milk, and the better suckling empties the breast more fully. An empty breast tells the brain to make more milk. An at-breast supplementer consists of a feeding tube placed at mother's nipple, which delivers expressed milk or formula from a bag or bottle around mother's neck to the baby as he is nursing. See Chapter 13, Supplementation, for more information on at-breast supplementers.

*Guidelines for Use*

| **Step 1: Preparing Your Breasts for Making Milk** |
| --- |
| Not applicable because baby hasn't arrived yet. |
| **Step 2: Starting to Make Milk** |
| Not applicable because baby hasn't arrived yet. |
| **Step 3: Breastfeeding and Making More Milk** |
| As always with breastfeeding, feed according to baby's cues. For most mothers who induce lactation, nursing at least 10 to 12 times per day is optimal. Less frequently may result in more supplementation. Much more frequently can be overwhelming for mother.<br><br>If baby is interested in nursing less frequently than 8 or 9 times per day and you are supplementing with expressed milk or formula, consider decreasing the amount you are supplementing at each feeding. Baby will likely be interested in breastfeeding more often, and ultimately taking less supplemental milk or formula. (See Chapter 13 for more information on supplementation.) |

## My Story: Breastfeeding Rosa FREQUENTLY

*In breastfeeding both my biological babies and my adopted baby, I breastfed them whenever they cued me that they needed to nurse. For my biological babies, this amounted to nursing eight or nine times per day, right in line with what most of the breastfeeding literature suggests breastfed babies typically do. When Rosa, my adopted baby, seemed to nurse all the time, I started keeping a log. Fourteen times per day! Based on the research I've done for this book, I now understand that breastfeeding generally needs to be more frequent when lactation is induced. Is it because the mother's breast tissue doesn't develop as fully when there isn't pregnancy? Is it because babies who were birthed by another mother need more of the bonding that breastfeeding offers? I would guess both are true. In the end, I decided that breastfeeding 14 times per day (which is more than is even typical for adopted babies) was still better for us than the alternative, which would be have been supplementation, and possibly a less-content baby. It was very challenging to nurse this often, but I wouldn't have traded it for the world!*

## Breastfeeding for Comfort Only

For mothers who are not concerned with producing a significant quantity of milk, the breast can still be used for comforting baby, much as we use a pacifier in our culture today. It is an excellent way to bond with your baby!

When babies suckle for comfort, they tend to suckle in a different way than suckling for nourishment. The baby's suckle tends to be quicker and with less suction, like a flutter, than when the baby suckles for nourishment. As a result, this type of breastfeeding may be less effective in increasing in milk production.

Many babies won't be interested in the breast without the flow of milk, but some will. Some babies will be interested for a while, but wean earlier than they might have if milk was flowing. One way to avoid this risk is to supplement with an at-breast supplementer, if that is something you are comfortable doing.

### Michaela's Story:  Breastfeeding for Comfort Only

*When baby Eva arrived, Michaela had been pumping only droplets of milk. Michaela decided to stop pumping when Eva arrived, because she wanted to focus on being with Eva instead of being with the breast pump. Michaela offered Eva formula from a bottle, and ended the feeding by comforting Eva at the breast. Michaela enjoyed the closeness that she felt with Eva at this time, and Eva seemed to enjoy it very much too!*

# Pumping

Pumping is the most efficient way to regularly stimulate your breasts and remove milk.  You will get the best results when you choose the right type of pump. A double-electric breast pump has attachments for pumping both breasts at the same time, and it cycles using electricity rather than by hand. Choose a double-electric breast pump FDA approved for multiple users. This type of pump is sturdy enough for frequent, long-term use, and is effective enough to establish and increase milk production. A list of breast pumps appropriate for inducing lactation is available on the Products, page of my website. Although these types of pumps can be very expensive, they are often available for rental. See Appendix A, Tips for Pumping Success, for suggestions on how to find a reliable source for renting your breast pump and for numerous other ideas for getting the best results from your breast pump.

## Remi's Story: Remi goes on a "Pumping Holiday"

*While Remi was waiting to adopt her son from Guatemala, she pumped about eight times per day—except for the days when she went on a "pumping holiday." After she started producing milk in Step 2, once or twice a month, for two to three months, Remi would spend her days off work doing nothing except eating, drinking, watching TV, and pumping. During those days, she would pump until she could not get any more milk from the pump, rest for 30 to 60 minutes, and then pump again. By the time she met her son, Remi was producing 24 ounces per day!*

A mother can continue to use her pump after her baby has arrived and is breastfeeding well. Continuing to pump after baby arrives is a very personal choice. Certainly, it is an effective method of boosting milk production, but it is time away from your precious little one. Some mothers are ready to pack up the breast pump when baby arrives (at least until they return to work), others will keep it around to pump whenever the time is right, while others will continue to pump frequently throughout the day (and sometimes night).

### Power Pumping

Power Pumping, a pumping technique developed by Catherine Watson Genna, IBCLC, and Kate Sharp, IBCLC, is an effective way of boosting milk production for busy breastfeeding mothers. It is a similar concept to the "pumping holiday" described above, but it is designed for mothers who are also caring for their breastfeeding baby, as in Step 3. It mimics the frequency days when babies breastfeed more often than normal in order to increase their mother's milk production when they are going through a growth spurt. Genna and Sharp suggest that a mother place the breast pump in a location that she passes by frequently throughout the day. Then, each time the mother passes by the pump or has a few minutes, she pumps for five to ten minutes. A mother can pump as frequently as every 45 minutes. Genna and Sharp recommend power pumping for just a few days at a time. Days when both mother and partner are home or when extra help is available are good choices (Genna, 2009).

## Pumping with Breast Massage

Including breast massage in your pumping routine can significantly improve your output from the breast pump (Morton, 2012). It also increases the fat content in your milk by helping to release the more viscous hindmilk (Lee, 2011). Massage one breast at a time while pumping by holding the kit with one hand and massaging the breast with the other hand, or use a hands-free bra to massage both breasts at the same time. Massage the breast with kneading or small circular motions as described in the breast massage section below, or compress the breast by firmly squeezing your breast between your thumb and the remaining fingers. If you notice a firm, full area on the breast, give some extra attention to massaging that area.

Another approach to pumping with breast massage is to pump until the milk flow slows down, then massage to bring on another milk ejection (let-down), and pump again until the flow stops. One popular way to massage to assist a milk ejection, developed by Chele Marmet, is the massage, stroke, shake. Massage your breasts as described below. Then stroke your breasts by lightly raking your fingernails from the chest wall toward the nipple. Finally, lean forward so that your nipples face the floor and gently shake your breasts (Marmet, 2001).

### Pumping with Hand Expression

In addition to breast massage, hand expression has also been found to significantly increase output from the breast pump (Morton, 2012). After pumping as suggested above, tip the flanges so that they function as a funnel and hand express (as explained below) directly into the flanges of your breast pump. Even if you are able to express very little milk, hand expression is an excellent way to stimulate your breasts to boost your production.

## Hand Expression

Hand expression is the original "breast pump!" While it is generally not as efficient as a double-electric breast pump, it has many advantages. It is free and convenient: it does not require special equipment or an electrical outlet. Mothers who hand express have better long-term breastfeeding outcomes, particularly first-time mothers (Auerbach & Avery, 1981). One reason for this may be that hand expression increases a mother's comfort and confidence in her breasts' ability to nourish and nurture her baby.

Hand expression involves compressing the areola (the dark area around the nipple) with your fingers in order to stimulate the nipples and eventually release milk from the breasts. Dr. Jane Morton (2010) at Stanford University then suggests that the mother place her thumb and forefinger around the breasts about an inch behind the base of her nipple, and press, compress, release:

1. Press the fingers toward the chest wall, being careful not

to pull the skin.

2. Compress the fingers toward each other.

3. Release the fingers by relaxing all pressure on the breast.

Dr. Morton has some helpful video demonstrations of hand expression that you can connect to on my Links page.

Hand expression can be used in Step 2, when mother has started to make milk. It is much more time consuming than double pumping (pumping both breasts at the same time); however, some mothers find they have better results with hand expression than with a breast pump. You will likely need a receptacle for your expressed milk: a wide-mouthed container, such as a coffee mug, works great. Since you will need one hand for expressing, and the other for holding the receptacle, alternating breasts every few minutes helps to get more milk, and it gives tired fingers on each hand a rest. One option is to split hand-expression sessions with double-pumping sessions, spending more time with hand expression at the beginning when you are producing small quantities, and gradually shifting towards more time pumping as your volume increases.

In Step 3, hand expression is another option for continuing to increase milk production after baby has arrived. Some mothers find hand expression easier to manage than pumping once they are breastfeeding frequently. Hand express after or between breastfeeding. You can hand express whenever and wherever you have a few minutes and some privacy: nothing needs to be assembled and disassembled, no parts require special cleaning, and there is no need for an outlet. Some mothers will hand express for a few minutes every time they go to the bathroom, and after taking a shower. The warm water streaming onto your breasts in the shower is an excellent breast massage before hand expressing!

*Guidelines for Use*

| |
|---|
| **Step 1: Preparing Your Breasts for Making Milk** |
| Not recommended |
| **Step 2: Starting to Make Milk** |
| Begin pumping your breasts with low suction for no more than 5 minutes, 8-10 times per day. After about one week, gently raise the suction level and increase pumping time to at least 15 minutes. Once you are producing milk, continue your pumping session as long as you are getting milk. Make sure one of those pumping times is in the middle of the night. Some mothers find that drinking a large glass of water just before bedtime will set off their natural alarm clock during a time of light sleep. While it is not a good idea to have large stretches of time without pumping, it is not essential that pumping sessions be equally spaced throughout the day. Babies breastfeed in clusters, and you can pump in clusters. Continue for about six weeks, or until baby is breastfeeding. |
| **Step 3: Breastfeeding and Making More Milk** |
| As needed to increase milk production. Pump 10 minutes after or between breastfeeding as mother is able. |

(Marmet, 2001)


**Hand Expression with Breast Massage**

Breast massage is highly recommended whenever you do hand expression. Just as breast massage increases the output from pumping, it also increases the output from hand expression—and it is even more convenient since your hands are already on your breasts. Massage your breasts before hand expressing, or in the middle of your session. Chele Marmet developed the massage-stroke-shake technique specifically for hand expression. She suggests hand expressing until the flow of milk slows down, then massage, stroke, shake to assist another milk ejection, then express again. The process can be repeated for a total of 20 to 30 minutes (Marmet, 2001).

*Guidelines for Use*

| Step 1:  Preparing Your Breasts for Making Milk |
| --- |
| Not recommended |
| **Step 2:  Starting to Make Milk** |
| 8 to 10 times per day for up to 20 to 30 minutes for about six weeks, or until baby is breastfeeding.  If you are splitting pumping sessions and hand-expression sessions, then they can combine for 8 to 10 times per day.  If you are combining hand expression with pumping, the combined time is 20 to 30 minutes. |
| **Step 3:  Breastfeeding and Making More Milk** |
| As needed to increase milk production.  Hand express 10 minutes or less, after or between breastfeeding as mother is able. |

# Breast Massage

Breast massage is a quick and simple way to awaken your breasts to make milk. It is also a way of becoming familiar with your breasts, growing more comfortable and confident with their feel and function. If you wish, you can apply a warm compress to your breasts, such as a warm, moist washcloth. Then, massage the entire breast, either kneading by rolling your knuckles from the chest wall towards the nipples or pressing down in small circular motions (as in a breast cancer self-examination), spiraling from the chest wall toward the nipple.

*Guidelines for Use*

| **Step 1: Preparing Your Breasts for Making Milk** |
|---|
| 10 minutes, 8 to 10 times per day, for two weeks or more |
| **Step 2: Starting to Make Milk** |
| As desired with pumping or hand expression. |
| **Step 3: Breastfeeding and Making More Milk** |
| As desired with pumping or hand expression. |

## Nipple Manipulation

Nipple manipulation can help with breastfeeding without birthing in more than one way. It can help drive milk production by stimulating the hormones of lactation. It can also help the baby to latch by drawing out the nipples. Roll the nipple between your thumb and forefinger. Gently pull out on the nipple. Stroke the nipple. See my Links page for a demonstration of nipple manipulation with hand expression.

*Guidelines for Use*

| **Step 1: Preparing Your Breasts for Making Milk** |
|---|
| Up to 10 minutes, 8 to 10 times per day, for two weeks or more |
| **Step 2: Starting to Make Milk** |
| As desired with hand expression and breast massage. |
| **Step 3: Breastfeeding and Making More Milk** |
| As desired with hand expression and breast massage. |

## Partner Stimulation

Just as a typical breastfeeding situation arises out of sexual intimacy with a partner, yours can too. Partners can participate in several of the physical techniques described above: massaging mother's breasts, manipulating her nipples, and hand expressing. The partner can also suckle from mother's breasts in order to prepare her breasts for making milk. Jimmie Lynne Avery reported the following from her research on adoptive mothers who induced lactation.

> Many couples noted that assistance from the [partner] with breast massage and manual expression, as well as suckling by the [partner], seemed to create a close bond between them prior to adoption. This is similar to experience described by couples participating in prenatal childbirth classes and exercises in which the [partner] has an active role in birth preparations and delivery (accessed July 3, 2012).

### Guidelines for Use

| Step 1: Preparing Your Breasts for Making Milk |
| --- |
| 10 minutes, as often as desired, for two weeks or more |
| Step 2: Starting to Make Milk |
| Not typically done in this step, but couldn't hurt. |
| Step 3: Breastfeeding and Making More Milk |
| Not typically done in this step, but couldn't hurt. |

# Chapter 12

# MEDICATIONS FOR
# INDUCING LACTATION

## Galactogogues

As emphasized in the previous chapters, physical techniques in which the breasts are frequently and effectively stimulated and emptied are the only necessary methods for inducing lactation. However, medications—either pharmaceutical or herbal—can significantly boost the effectiveness of the physical techniques. Medications and foods that help increase milk production are often referred to as galactogogues. Several of the protocols described in Chapter 10, Approaches to Inducing Lactation, may have a galactogogue medication component to them in addition to the physical techniques. As with any medication—either pharmaceutical or herbal—consult with your doctor before using. Medications may have potentially dangerous side effects or may interact with other medications you are taking.

## Pharmaceuticals

Medications can play a helpful role in inducing lactation. In Step 1, they can be used to simulate the hormonal changes that occur with pregnancy to prepare the breasts for breastfeeding. During pregnancy, the hormones estrogen, progesterone, and prolactin increase. Together these hormones build milk ducts and glandular breast tissue. Estrogen and progesterone can be boosted with the use of a birth control pill, or progesterone and goat's rue (an herbal medication). Alternately, progesterone levels alone can be boosted with a progesterone medication (although this is likely to be less effective than the birth control pill). Prolactin is increased with the medication Domperidone.

In Steps 2 and 3, the breasts begin to produce milk. Estrogen and progesterone levels must drop. While these hormones are very helpful in developing breast tissue, they also suppress milk production. Domperidone, on the other hand, can continue to be helpful in Steps 2 and 3 since prolactin is the hormone responsible for milk production.

## Birth Control Pill

The birth control pill (BCP) is a balanced combination of estrogen and progestin (synthetic progesterone), which can be taken to build milk ducts and glandular breast tissue, as typically occurs in pregnancy to prepare the breasts for lactation. The estrogen and progesterone levels achieved with the birth control pill are minute compared to those achieved during pregnancy: building breast tissue doesn't require the level of these hormones that sustaining a pregnancy does. As one mother remarked, "It seemed quite strange to be taking [the birth control pill] not to prevent having a baby, but in order to provide for one" (Koning, 2011).

*Guidelines for Use*

## Step 1: Preparing Your Breasts for Making Milk

Choose a monophasic BCP at containing at most 0.035 mg of estrogen and at least 1 mg of progestin. Options include the following: Demulen 1/35, Microgestin 1.5/30, Necon 1/35, Norethin 1/35E, Norinyl 1+35, Nortrel 1/35, Ortho 1/35, Ortho-Novum 1/35, Zovia 1/35 (Newman & Goldfarb, accessed July 11, 2012). Because you are taking the BCP for developing breast tissue and not for contraception, you can begin taking it anytime during your menstrual cycle. Take one "active" pill each day (skipping the week of placebo) for a minimum of two months. Continuing to take the BCP for six to nine months will increase its effectiveness since this is how long it takes a mother's breast tissue to fully develop in pregnancy (Newman & Goldfarb, accessed October 26, 2012).

## Step 2: Starting to Make Milk

Not recommended.

## Step 3: Breastfeeding and Making More Milk

Not recommended.

Getting insurance reimbursement for the BCP can be a little tricky because you will be going through a month's worth of pills in three weeks' time by skipping the week of placebo. Check your policy. My pharmacist was able to help me time my prescriptions to the day in order to get reimbursement.

### Alexis's Story

*Alexis was very experienced with using medications to boost her progesterone and estrogen levels as part of her past fertility treatments. She knew that these medications offered much higher dosages of estrogen*

171

*and progesterone than the birth control pill. So with her fertility doctor's guidance, Alexis used her old fertility medications for two months instead of the birth control pill in Step 1. Alexis attributes her full milk supply after such a short Step 1 to the use of these heavy-duty hormones.*

## Progesterone

Progesterone is an alternative to the birth control pill for mothers who cannot or choose not to take a birth control pill.[1] This form of progesterone is not a birth control pill—the recommended progesterone medications are those used for menstrual or fertility difficulties. Progesterone is not likely to result in as much milk production as with the birth control pill (Jack Newman, MD, personal communication, December 15, 2012).

> **Perspectives on Taking the Birth Control Pill without Placebo**
>
> Taking a birth control pill without a week of placebo is not an idea exclusive to inducing lactation. Women have been doing this for years in order to eliminate their periods if they have experienced endometriosis, menstrual migraines, severe menstrual pain or moodiness, or other undesirable effects of menstruation. More recently, women are choosing to eliminate their periods simply for convenience. One woman reported that she has not menstruated for 10 years while on the BCP continuously. While there hasn't been research into the safety of this, no adverse effects have been reported (Kam, 2008).

[1] Estrogen and progestin birth control pills are associated with greater health risks for women over the age of 35.

Until recent times, it was typical for mothers to have only one or two periods in nine to 24 months, because they breastfed for two or more years. Because of this natural time of amenorrhea that breastfeeding mothers experience, some physicians have speculated that suppressing cycles with a continuous active birth control pill for a year or more is not unreasonable nor unsafe (C. Vlastos, MD, personal communication, September 20, 2012).

## Guidelines for Use

**Step 1: Preparing Your Breasts for Making Milk**

Prometrium 100 mg (natural progesterone) or Provera 2.5 mg (progestin) once per day for a minimum of two months. Continuing to take the progesterone for six to nine months will increase its effectiveness as this is how long it takes a mother's breast tissue to fully develop in pregnancy. (Progesterone creams are not recommended because they do not provide progesterone in a reliable manner.)

**Step 2: Starting to Make Milk**

Not recommended.

**Step 3: Breastfeeding and Making More Milk**

Not recommended.

### Domperidone

Domperidone is a medication developed to treat gastrointestinal issues. A fortunate side effect of this medication is a significant increase in the body's release of prolactin, the hormone responsible for milk production. Domperidone is the most effective medication for increasing milk production and is the safest pharmaceutical medication for this purpose (Gabay, 2002). Domperidone can be taken along with the birth control pill to mimic the hormonal changes that occur during pregnancy, as well as once you start to produce milk. See Appendix B, Domperidone: "The Ideal Galactogogue," for more information about this medication and the Products, page of my website for information on how to obtain it.

### *Guidelines for Use*

| Step 1: Preparing Your Breasts for Making Milk |
| --- |
| 20mg 4x/day. Some mothers have safely taken up to 40mg 4x/day (J. Newman, MD, personal communication, December 16, 2012). Take this medication 30 minutes before a meal for best absorption. |
| **Step 2: Starting to Make Milk** |
| 20mg 4x/day. Some mothers have safely taken up to 40mg 4x/day (J. Newman, MD, personal communication, December 16, 2012). Take this medication 30 minutes before a meal for best absorption. |
| **Step 3: Breastfeeding and Making More Milk** |
| 20mg 4x/day. Some mothers have safely taken up to 40mg 4x/day (J. Newman, MD, personal communication, December 16, 2012). Take this medication 30 minutes before a meal for best absorption. |

### Remi's Story: Domperidone Does the Trick

*We heard from Remi, who went on a pumping holiday, in the last chapter. Remi elected to skip Step 1, and started inducing lactation in Step 2 by pumping and taking herbal medications. For several months, she continued pumping with no milk output. At that point, she decided to add Domperidone into her Step 2 plan and started making milk within a few days.*

## "I Want to go Natural"

I have heard this from many mothers-to-be. Instead of the medications above, they will choose herbal medications, or no medications at all. It makes sense, doesn't it? We are choosing to breastfeed in part because it is natural. It is important to consider, though, that mothers who do not use pharmaceuticals are likely to need to supplement more with formula, a product that is not natural. There is a tradeoff.

# Herbs

Although suggested dosages of medications are provided (see above), dosages for herbal medications are not. Potency of herbal medications is not standardized and varies greatly according to the form of the herb and its quality. Herbal supplements come in the form of a tincture, dried capsules, or tea. A tincture is the most potent form of an herb. Tinctures are available as a liquid or in liquid capsules. The liquid form is somewhat less expensive and tends to be absorbed more quickly than the liquid capsules, but it has a strong, unpleasant taste. Many mothers prefer the convenience and lack of taste of the liquid capsule. Tea is the least potent form of herbs. While some mothers who breastfeed babies by birth find teas helpful in increasing milk production, mothers who induce lactation tend to require herbs in a more potent form (S. Cox, Motherlove Herbals, personal communication, November 28, 2012). In order to be effective, your herbal medication should be fresh and of good quality: herbs in dried or tea form should smell fragrant and be distinct in color (Jacobson, 2007). Start out with the recommended dosages on the product and adjust from there as needed. Herbs should be taken before meals.

One recommended way to use herbal galactogogues is to rotate them. When a mother takes a particular herbal galactogogue for a period of time, it may lose its effectiveness. Either discontinuing an herb (or combination of herbs) for a couple of weeks and then reintroducing it, or switching herbal galactogogues periodically can improve results. Contact your local herbalist or lactation consultant familiar with herbs for additional guidance.

Any medication, whether herbal or pharmaceutical, that is strong enough to cause a desirable effect on the body also has the potential to cause negative side effects. Regardless of popularity and easy availability, herbs should always be used with caution. Before using any herbal galactogogue, see Appendix C, Potential Side Effects and Safety Cautions for Herbal Galactogogues.

The information below regarding these herbs was compiled from *The Nursing Mother's Herbal* (Humphrey, 2003), *Motherfood* (Jacobson, 2007), and *The Breastfeeding Mother's Guide to Making More Milk* (West & Marasco, 2009). For more information on these herbs, please refer to any of these excellent resources.

### *Guidelines for Use (all herbal galactogogues)*

| **Step 1: Preparing Your Breasts for Making Milk** |
| --- |
| Goat's rue only: use according to package directions and adjust as needed. No other herbs are suggested during this step. |
| **Step 2: Starting to Make Milk** |
| Use according to package directions and adjust as needed. |
| **Step 3: Breastfeeding and Making More Milk** |
| Use according to package directions and adjust as needed. |

## Alfalfa

Alfalfa, when used as a galactogogue, is generally taken in combination with other herbal galactogogues. Alfalfa supports the function of the pituitary gland, which secretes the lactation hormones prolactin and oxytocin. It may also help to develop breast tissue.

## Blessed Thistle

Although blessed thistle is considered a mild galactogogue by itself, it is generally used in combination with fenugreek. The combination of fenugreek and blessed thistle is believed to increase the effectiveness of either used separately.

## Fennel

Fennel is another herb reputed to build breast tissue. It may also aid milk ejection.

## Fenugreek

Fenugreek is the most commonly used herbal galactogogue in the United States today. It helps to increase milk production by increasing prolactin levels. It is a relative of goat's rue and is also reputed to help build breast tissue.

## Goat's Rue

Goat's rue is the only herbal galactogogue suggested during Step 1. Although many of the herbs recommended for inducing lactation are reputed to help build glandular breast tissue, goat's rue has the strongest reputation in this area. It can be used on its own in Step 1 or in combination with a progesterone medication (see above). Goat's rue is a phytoestrogen, a chemical found in plants that acts like estrogen in the body. When it is taken in combination with progesterone, it creates a combination of estrogen and progesterone as with the birth control pill[2]. When used alone, goat's rue's impact on breast tissue development may not be as strong as when taken with progesterone, but most mothers will still notice significant breast changes in about two weeks. Goat's rue can be especially helpful for mothers with polycystic ovarian syndrome (PCOS).

**Saw Palmetto**

Saw Palmetto is another herb believed to build glandular breast tissue. It may increase the quantity and fat content of milk, and is particularly helpful for mothers with polycystic ovarian syndrome (PCOS).

**Shatavari**

Shatavari is a popular herb in India and China used for enhancing fertility and lactation. Studies have shown it to increase glandular breast tissue and milk production in animals.

## Foods

Chapter 9, Making Milk: What to Expect, describes how a healthy diet sets the stage for healthy lactation. We can take this a step further. Many foods are considered lactogenic: these are particular foods, or groups of foods, with a long-standing reputation for increasing milk production. These foods are identified as lactogenic, not as a result of

[2] Goat's rue should not be taken with BCP because it throws off the balance of estrogen and progesterone (L. Goldfarb, personal communication, July 25, 2011).

scientific research, but as a result of cultural traditions. Consistently across cultures, foods reputed to increase milk production tend to be high in fiber and filled with vitamins, especially in nutrients B complex, iron, calcium, omega-3s, and zinc (Marasco, 2012). Some helpful lactogenic foods are listed below. See *Motherfood* by Hilary Jacobson (2007) for a more extensive listing of lactogenic foods as well as recipes that use them.

- **Whole Grains**. Whole grains, such as oats, brown rice, and barley, have longstanding reputations for increasing milk production. Avoid instant or quick-cooking grains as they are not as effective at boosting milk production as the unprocessed whole versions of the grains.

- **Dark Green Vegetables**. Eating dark green vegetables can support healthy milk production as well as supporting a healthy you. Some mothers have good results with "green drinks." (Avoid "green drinks" containing parsley because this herb can suppress milk production.)

- **Nuts and Seeds**. Almonds are the most lactogenic nut, but cashews and pecans can also be helpful. Sesame seeds and flaxseed are reported to be the most lactogenic seeds.

- **Malunggay**. The leaves of the malunggay tree, also known as the drumstick tree or moringa, are considered the most nutrient-rich on earth, as well as being very high in antioxidants. Malunggay has been consumed as part of a healthy diet and as a galactogogue in Asian countries for thousands of years. Several small studies have shown it to be effective in increasing milk production. It can sometimes be found fresh in ethnic grocery stores, or it can be purchased in a dried form. The fresh leaves can be prepared and used like spinach.

179

See my Products, page to obtain dried malunggay, or search the Internet for malunggay or moringa (D. West, personal communication, February 19, 2013).

- **Coconut Milk.** Traditional cultures, such as those found in New Guinea, Zulu tribes in Africa, aboriginal communities in Australia, and Tierra del Fuego in South America, have used the same general techniques for inducing lactation: breast-feeding, breast massage, and drinking coconut milk (Biervliet et al., 2001; Moran & Gilad, 2007). It is hypothesized that coconut milk may be popular as a lactogenic food because it is white and creamy, just like mother's milk (Jacobson, 2007; World Health Organization, 1998).

Pharmaceuticals, herbs, or foods may play a significant role in the amount of milk you are able to produce. As a result, these galacto-gogues may be an important part of your breastfeeding plan, or you may choose not to take galactogogues beyond eating a balanced diet of whole foods. Using the protocols in Chapter 10 as a guide, you can find the right combination of galactogogues for you.

# Chapter 13

# SUPPLEMENTATION

Supplementation refers to providing your baby with food other than the milk directly from your breasts. As I've mentioned throughout this book, most mothers who induce lactation need to supplement breastfeeding because they are not able to produce enough milk each day to meet their babies' daily intake needs. This chapter will help you make the most of breastfeeding while ensuring that your baby is getting enough nourishment via supplementation.

## What to Supplement With

According to the World Health Organization (WHO), breastfeeding is the first choice for feeding a baby. You are reading this book because it is also your first choice to nurture and nourish your baby from your breasts. If you are inducing lactation, it is likely you will have to supplement the milk your baby receives from breastfeeding with nourishment from another source. For babies under six months of age, the WHO has recommended the following options (WHO, 2003):

1st choice:  Breastfeeding
2nd choice:  Mother's own expressed milk

3rd choice:     Another mother's milk

4th choice:     Infant formula

For babies older than six months, solid foods can be added to supplement breastfeeding. Many mothers who induce lactation will feed their babies a combination of these options. If you are combining milk (either your own expressed milk or another mother's milk) with formula, don't mix the milk with formula. Always feed the baby human milk first, then feed with formula if needed. This way, you are less likely to end up discarding the precious milk.

## Mother's Own Expressed Milk

A mother who has pumped or hand expressed her own milk can give that milk to her baby at a later time. Mothers who induce lactation may have milk stored from pumping or hand expressing before their baby arrived. Some mothers choose to continue pumping or hand expressing once their baby has arrived to further stimulate milk production. In both cases, this "liquid gold" has not only helped them to produce milk for breastfeeding their baby, but is has provided the best supplement available for their baby.

## Kim's Story: Supplementing Twins with her Own Expressed Milk

*By the time Kim's twins were born via surrogacy, she was pumping more than 15 ounces per day. While Kim originally hoped to produce "at least some drops" of milk for her babies, her pumping success motivated her to change her goal. Her new goal was to feed her babies exclusively with her own milk for their first month of life: a combination of the milk the babies received while breastfeeding, and the milk she pumped before and after they arrived. Kim met her goal!*

## Debra's Story:  Sharing Milk with Big Brother

*Debra had been hoping to breastfeed her adopted baby. Just three days before she was matched with newborn baby Travis, Debra learned that she was pregnant. Due to medications she was taking to sustain the pregnancy, her doctor advised that she not try to induce lactation. However, when Debra gave birth to baby Edwin when Travis was eight months old, Edwin shared some of his milk with his older brother!*

## Another Mother's Milk

When a mother's own milk cannot meet her baby's nutritional needs, she may choose to feed her baby with another mother's milk. In the case of surrogacy, your gestational carrier may be willing to express milk for a period of time for your baby. This is something to consider when searching for a surrogate and can be included in your pre-birth order. If she is amenable to this, you are very lucky! For most mothers who are inducing lactation, obtaining another mother's milk is a bit trickier.

Some breastfeeding-without-birthing mothers are able to obtain donated milk from a nonprofit milk bank. The mothers who donate milk to nonprofit milk banks are thoroughly screened for diseases and medications, alcohol, and nicotine that may be dangerous to baby when passed into the milk. Once received at the milk-banking facility, the milk is processed under sterile conditions, pasteurized, and finally tested for bacterial growth before being released. The Links page of my website can connect you with the Human Milk Banking Association of North America, where you can find more information about donor milk and locate a local nonprofit milk bank. Be prepared, however, to face some obstacles in the process. Your local nonprofit milk bank may be reserving its limited stock for ill or preterm infants. Due to extensive screening and processing, the milk is likely to be extremely expensive ($3.00 to $4.50 USD an ounce). Additionally, if your baby is not hospitalized, you will need a prescription from your pediatrician.

If obtaining milk from a nonprofit milk bank is not possible, donated milk can still be a viable option for you: mothers have always quietly, informally received donated milk from family members and friends.

> When my sister and brother-in-law adopted my nephew from Korea, there was no question where he would get his milk: from me! I was breastfeeding my daughter at the time, and I began pumping and freezing extra milk for him about eight weeks before they were due to pick him up. I continued pumping milk for him for eight months (Granju & Kennedy, 1999, p. 99).

Recently, some other options have become available. Though not milk banks, there are online sources of milk sharing: mothers producing extra milk donate their milk to others in need and they connect with each other via the Internet. These donor mothers don't get paid, but they may get reimbursed for storage, shipping, and other expenses incurred. Unlike the milk banks, however, these donors are not screened, the milk is not pasteurized, and the handling and storage of the milk is not monitored. As a result, it is essential to take precautions whenever accepting donated milk. Let's take a close look at the concerns regarding milk sharing and how you can minimize the risks involved.

## Safety Practices for Milk Sharing[1]

| |
|---|
| *Risk: Dangerous illnesses can be passed from the donor mother to baby through shared milk.* |
| **Step 1: Assess Risks** |
| HIV and HTLV (1 and 2) are the only dangerous illnesses that can be passed to babies through donated milk. Both are very rare in the U.S. among mothers who donate milk.[2] |
| **Step 2: Screen Donor** |
| Donors can be screened with a blood test for HIV and HTLV.[3] |
| **Step 3: Treat Milk** |
| In the case of positive test results or as an extra precaution, HTLV can be inactivated by freezing and HIV can be inactivated by flash heating (Gribble & Hausman, 2012). |
| **Consider the Alternative** |
| Formula does not contain the immunological properties of human milk that protect babies against every illness. |

[1]Please note that the recommendations presented here for managing the risks of milk sharing do not apply to preterm or babies hospitalized for other reasons. In these cases, consider donor milk from a nonprofit human milk bank your first choice.

[2]While many dangerous diseases can pass into the milk, only a few can actually infect a healthy full-term baby who drinks the milk. The few exceptions are Human Immunodeficiency Virus (HIV) and Human T-Cell Leukemia Viruses (HTLV1 and 2). Although HIV and HLTV can be transmitted via human milk, they are not easily transmitted; only through repeated exposure over a long period of time will a baby contract these diseases through human milk (Gribble & Hausman, 2012). This is unlike receiving infected blood during a blood transfusion, which has a very high rate of infection.

HIV or HTLV contaminated human milk is very rare in the United States. According to one recent study of milk bank donors, 0.37% of donors screened positive for HIV and 0.55% screened positive for HTLV. These numbers may be inflated estimates of actual milk contamination, because blood screening tests yield a high proportion of false positives (Cohen et al., 2009).

[3]Donor screening is not fail-safe: an infected person will not test positive for HIV for several weeks after being infected, because it takes this long for the HIV antibodies to be detectible with screening tests. Mothers are also encouraged to screen potential donors for behaviors that may make them higher risk for HIV: risky sexual behaviors, intravenous drug use, or a recent blood transfusion. In addition to HIV and HTLV, the Human Milk Banking Association of North America also recommends screening for Hepatitis B, Hepatitis C, and Syphilis. However, neither the American Academy of Pediatrics (AAP) nor the Center for Disease Control (CDC) considers these diseases contraindications to breastfeeding.

| *Risk: Shared milk can be contaminated with unhealthy bacteria.* |
|---|
| **Step 1: Assess Risks** |
| All expressed milk contains bacteria, most of which is not dangerous. Human milk also contains anti-bacterial properties.[1] |
| **Step 2: Screen Donor** |
| See sidebar below for guidelines regarding the safety recommendations for the handling and storage of human milk. Any potential donor can be asked to comply with these procedures. |
| **Step 3: Treat Milk** |
| Flash heating destroys the majority of bacteria in human milk yet maintains the anti-bacterial properties of the milk (Isreal-Ballard et al., 2006). |
| **Consider the Alternative** |
| Bacteria found in formula have caused infants to contract enterobacter sakazakii, salmonellosis, meningitis, bacteremia, necrotizing enterocolitis, and encephalitis. |

[1]Any time milk is expressed, it contains bacteria. Usually this bacterium is normal skin flora and not at all dangerous (Gribble & Hausman, 2012). However, the donor mother can pass certain pathogenic bacteria, such as Salmonella ssp., Group B Streptococcus, or Listeria through her milk. Rarely have infants been infected with these bacteria via human milk (May, 1999). Shared human milk may also contain bacteria due to unhygienic handling and storage practices. It is not clear that even these bacteria are harmful to infants (Gribble & Hausman, 2012). Fortunately, human milk also contains anti-bacterial properties: it is resistant to the growth of bacteria.

*Risk: Medications taken by the donor mother can be passed to your baby through her milk.*

### Step 1: Assess Risks

When a mother takes any medication, the amount of the medication in mother's milk is very small, usually <1% of the mother's dosage, and in most cases is considered safe for the baby (Hale, 2012).[2]

### Step 2: Screen Donor

Any potential milk donor should share which medications that she is taking along with the dosage of each medication.[3]

### Step 3: Treat Milk

### Consider the Alternative

Formula containing melamine caused hundreds of thousands of babies in China to become seriously ill, and some of the babies died. Formula has also been found to contain pesticides, PVC plastic, glass particles, and beetle body parts.

[2]Remember, any mother who is donating milk is also feeding her own baby the same milk.

[3]Any potential milk donor should share which medications, including prescription, over-the-counter, vitamins, supplements or herbs that she is taking along with the dosage of each medication. Nicotine (from smoking) and alcohol are also considered drugs. Any medications that the donor mother is taking can be researched by a lactation consultant or other health professional with access to the most recent edition of *Medications & Mother's Milk* by Thomas Hale, Ph.D. This publication contains the most comprehensive information regarding the safety of milk when mother is taking a particular medication.

### Flash Heating of Human Milk

Flash heating donated milk can inactivate diseases and destroy bacteria passed into human milk, while retaining most of the milk's nutrition, antibodies, and antimicrobial properties. Flash heating is different than flash pasteurization, which requires specialized equipment not compatible with home use. Flash heating is a simple technique using readily available materials in which the milk is heated very hot, but for a very short time (Yang, 2007).

### *How to Flash Heat*

Put donated milk into a glass bottle or jar and place it in an aluminum pot filled with water. Heat the pot over a high flame. As soon as the water is boiling, remove the jar or bottle of milk. See the Links page on my website to view a video demonstration of flash heating.

Milk sharing can be a comparatively safe way to meet your baby's nutritional and immunological needs. Consistent with recommendations set by the World Health Organization, donor milk is generally considerably safer than infant formula. When done safely, milk sharing can be a beautiful way parents can join together in community to support each other. See the Links page of my website for a listing of online resources for peer-to-peer milk sharing.

## Bethany's Story: Baby Linn's Milk Mama

*Bethany adopted baby Linn from Korea when Linn was six months old. While Bethany was able to provide some of her own milk for baby Linn, the rest of Linn's nourishment came from donated milk. Through a friend, Bethany connected with another mother who was already donating her expressed milk to two other babies. Combining Bethany's milk with that of her "Milk Mama," Linn exclusively drank human milk until she was 11 months old.*

## Wendy's Story: A Commitment to Human Milk for her Baby

*Wendy is an intended mother who was determined to exclusively feed her son Zander with human milk at her breast. She worked hard to induce lactation, and was able to produce enough milk to meet about one-third of Zander's nutritional needs. Wendy supplemented her milk supply with donated human milk fed to Zander at the breast using an at-breast supplementer. The milk was donated from various sources: a couple of personal contacts and numerous mothers she connected with through the milkshare.com networking website. Some of the donated milk was local, some was shipped frozen, and some Wendy was willing to drive up to two hours each way to pick up. When Wendy traveled across the country to visit family, and she decided to extend her stay beyond her original plans, she found a milk donor in the city she was visiting.*

## A Note on Milk Selling

Although the sale of human milk is legal in most states, it is fraught with ethical and safety issues. There is some concern that poor mothers will sell so much of their milk that there will not be enough for their own babies. Furthermore, milk selling is not monitored or regulated in any way (just as with peer-to-peer milk sharing). Because they are trying to make money, mothers selling human milk may not be motivated to be completely upfront regarding any medications, smoking or drinking habits, diet, or other potential negatives regarding their milk. They may also be tempted to boost the volume of their milk with water, cow's milk, infant formula, or another substance. It is not advisable for families to obtain human milk in this manner.

## Safe Handling and Storage of Human Milk

As a breastfeeding-without-birthing mother, you will likely need to supplement breastfeeding. Ideally, and in many cases, that supplement consists of expressed and stored human milk.

- Before your baby arrives, you may express your milk in order to establish milk production and to bank your milk for supplementation after baby arrives.
- After your baby arrives, you may express milk to build milk production and supplement breastfeeding.
- After your baby arrives, you may obtain milk from a donor mother who has expressed and stored her milk for the purpose of sharing it with another mother/baby pair.

If you are supplementing with human milk--your own or from another mother--make sure that the milk is handled and stored safely so as to prevent the growth of harmful bacteria. Even a healthy mother can provide unhealthy milk if she doesn't use good hygiene while pumping and storing her milk.

### *Handling of Human Milk*

Wash your hands before each pumping session. Wash your pump kit regularly in hot, soapy water; rinse; and then allow it to air dry. Although some guidelines suggest that the pump kit be washed after each use, another option would be to use the milk storage rules discussed below as your guideline for protecting your pump parts against bacterial growth: store pump parts at room temperature for four to six hours, and up to a day in the refrigerator in a zippered storage bag.

### Storage of Donated Milk

Milk-storage guidelines safeguard milk against unhealthy bacterial growth. The length of time milk must be stored determines where it must be stored: at room temperature, insulated cooler, refrigerator, or freezer. See the Links page of my website to access La Leche League's handy table of milk storage guidelines.

If you are pumping your milk for a baby who hasn't arrived yet, your expressed milk will most likely be stored in the freezer. Although milk can be frozen in small quantities, you will be producing such small quantities at first that you may need to accumulate the milk from several pumping sessions in order to fill a storage bag or bottle with even a couple of ounces. Cool freshly pumped milk in the refrigerator before adding it to frozen milk.

If you are receiving donated milk, how the donor mother should safely store her expressed milk depends upon how long the milk must be stored before it reaches you. Milk that is donated locally may be refrigerated or frozen depending upon when it will be picked up. Milk that is donated long distance must be frozen and shipped on dry ice.

**Infant Formula**

No one infant formula is universally recommended for supplementing a breastfed baby. A good place to start is the formula that your baby received if he was formula-fed before meeting you. Your pediatrician may also have a recommendation.

## How Much Human Milk or Formula Supplement is Needed?

Just like any breastfed baby, feed your baby according to his cues. If you are able to breastfeed your baby immediately after birth, you may not need to supplement breastfeeding even if you are not producing a lot of milk. During the first few days, a newborn baby requires an ounce or less of (mature) milk or formula per feeding. (We don't want to compare with a gestational mother who is breastfeeding because the colostrum she would be producing is much more calorie-rich than the mature milk that you will be producing.)

If you have started to produce milk before your baby arrives, you will have some idea how much you will need to supplement after those first few days: simply subtract the amount of milk your baby requires from the amount of milk you have been expressing each day. After the first few days of life, babies less than 10 pounds require approximately 2.5 ounces per pound per day. Babies over 10 pound, and at least four weeks old, will consume 25 to 32 ounces per day. But please don't get too caught up in these calculations–they are simply here as a starting guideline! Research data shows a huge range of milk intake for normal, healthy babies. Your baby is the expert on how much milk he needs.

Supplementation is a delicate balance. If too much supplemental human milk or formula is given, then baby takes less at the breast. If your baby is feeding less than eight or nine times per day, this may be an indication that you are supplementing more than necessary at each feeding. You may find that you are able to decrease the amount of supplement and breastfeed more often. On the other hand, if not enough supplement is given, then your baby won't be getting enough food. Watch for signs that your baby is not getting enough.

- **Poor weight gain.** A breastfed baby should regain his birth weight within 10 to 14 days. Breastfed babies should then gain weight as follows: 5 to 7 ounces per week for the first four months, 4 to 5 ounces per week when baby is four to six months old, and 2 to 4 ounces per week for the remainder of the first year. Pediatricians usually do a great job monitoring weight gain.

- **Less than three-to-five bowel movements per day during the newborn period.** Some exclusively breastfed babies older than four-to-six weeks stool infrequently, maybe once every few days.

- **Fussiness or excessive sleepiness after or between feedings.**

- **Test weights that indicate lower than anticipated milk transfer while breastfeeding.** Many lactation consultants in private practice have highly accurate baby scales designed to measure milk intake from breastfeeding. The lactation consultant can weigh the baby, then mother breastfeeds, and the baby is weighed again. When done properly, this technique is a fairly accurate measure of how many ounces the baby is taking in during a breastfeeding. That amount can be combined with the amount of supplement, if any, to determine whether baby is meeting his daily intake requirements.

## When to Offer the Supplement

Once you have determined about how much supplement your baby needs, if any, that amount must be divvied up throughout the day. Again, watch your baby's cues. Your baby will be hungrier at some feedings than others, just as us grown-ups have lighter meals, heavier meals, and snacks. Also, breastfeeding mothers make different amounts of milk throughout the day, so your baby may be getting more or less milk than average at a given feeding. With this in mind, a general guideline for supplementation is to divide the amount supplemented across most of the breastfeeding sessions. If your baby will tolerate a couple of breastfeeding sessions without supplementation each day, he will get used to the idea of breastfeeding without supplementation each time. If your baby is supplemented with a few larger amounts throughout the day (four ounces or more), then he may skip a breastfeeding session because he isn't hungry (Mohrbacher, 2010).

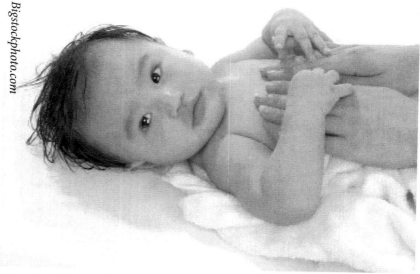

Massaging baby can help him gain more weight on less milk.

## Gaining More Weight on Less Milk

The most obvious way to decrease the amount of supplementation your baby needs is to continue to make more milk. Easier said than done, right? Another, more subtle, way to decrease the need to supplement is to decrease the amount of milk baby needs by helping him gain more weight on less milk.

- **Less Crying.** Crying is an aerobic activity. Less crying means fewer calories burned, thus reducing the amount of milk needed to grow (Lee, 2011). When parents respond sensitively and quickly to their baby's cues, they cry less. When parents practice the tools of latching and attaching in Chapter 6, their babies cry less.

- **Massage.** One study of preterm formula-fed babies showed that babies who received regular massages gained 47% more weight on the same amount of formula than the babies who did not receive massages (Field et al., 1986). To learn more about infant massage, check in your neighborhood for mommy-and-me massage classes, or see the Library page on my website.

## Weaning from the Supplement

A baby who is nursing well is the best stimulus for producing more milk. Hopefully, you will be able to gradually decrease the amount of supplement over time. Some mothers will eventually produce enough milk to exclusively breastfeed, but most will not. Some mothers find that they can breastfeed without supplementation at some feedings, even though they need to supplement at others. Often, mothers can eliminate the supplement during the middle of the night or first thing in the morning because milk production is naturally highest for all mothers during those times.

Eventually, all breastfeeding-without-birthing mothers will make enough milk so that their babies will no longer require supplementation, because all babies naturally wean from breastfeeding to eating solid foods. When your baby weans gradually by breastfeeding less and less, your milk production will eventually meet your baby's (decreasing) needs.

# How to Supplement

Whatever supplement you are providing for your baby—your expressed milk, donated milk, or infant formula—must be delivered to your baby using some sort of device. An at-breast supplementer allows a mother to continue breastfeeding while supplementing, and is the option I most recommend. It is not for everyone, and you may find another option, such as bottle-feeding, cup-feeding, or finger-feeding, that works better for you.

**At-Breast Supplementer**

An at-breast supplementer acts as an external milk duct carrying human milk or formula to mother's nipple through a tiny feeding tube. The feeding tube pulls human milk or formula from a bag or bottle that either hangs from mother's neck or rests close by. If you are not producing a significant amount of milk, and your baby refuses the breast unless milk is flowing, an at-breast supplementer may be your only option for your baby to breastfeed. If your baby will nurse without the flow of the supplementer, you may still find this device is your best choice.

196

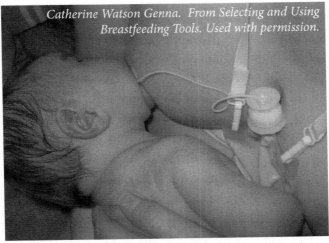

Catherine Watson Genna. From Selecting and Using Breastfeeding Tools. Used with permission.

This baby is being supplemented with the Lact-Aid at-breast supplementer. In this photo, the tube of the Lact-Aid is beneath a nipple shield that is holding it in place. For mothers who don't require a nipple shield, the tubing can also be held in place with surgical tape or a bandage with the adhesive strips trimmed from both sides of the gauze.

- **Your baby receives the supplement as he is nursing**. At-breast supplementation allows mother to completely feed at the breast, instead of partially breastfeeding and partially feeding from another device.

- **An at-breast supplementer stimulates more milk production**. Baby spends more time at the breast, providing extra physical stimulation. Also, the at-breast supplementer encourages more effective suckling because baby is encouraged by the ample flow of human milk or formula it provides.

- **A baby may lose interest in breastfeeding earlier without the reinforcement from a sufficient flow of human milk or formula.**

- **Using an at-breast supplementer allows mother to bond with her baby while breastfeeding even when she needs to supplement.**

197

| Lact-Aid | Supplemental Nursing System (SNS) |
|---|---|
| **Convenience** | |
| + Disposable bags minimize the number of parts to be cleaned.<br>+ Soft bag is much more comfortable against mother's chest.<br>+ Body heat can warm supplement in bag.<br>+ Because this device does not rely on gravity, mother can nurse in a variety of positions including laid-back and lying down.<br>- More complicated to assemble. | + Two feeding tubes eliminate the need to move tube from one side to the next.<br>+ Flow from the supplementer can be cut off so that baby can be latched with the feeding tube at the breast, but not receive a supplement until baby no longer actively suckling without supplement.<br>- Tube at breast from which baby is not breastfeeding can be an enticement for an older baby to play.<br>- Because the human milk or formula flows with gravity, the device will leak if not properly assembled.<br>- Because the human milk or formula flows with gravity, milk may continue to flow after baby has released the nipple. |
| **Cost** | |
| - Expensive<br>- Ongoing cost of purchasing disposable bags. | - Expensive |
| **Breastfeeding in Public** | |
| + Bag discreet under clothing.<br>- Feeding tube must be switched from one breast to the other. | - Hard bottle cannot be concealed under clothing. |
| **Impact on Milk Production** | |
| + More suction is required to pull supplement through tubing, better stimulating more milk production. | |

(West & Marasco, 2009)

Using an at-breast supplementer does have some disadvantages though. It is new to most mothers and takes some getting used to. Some smart little babies figure out where the flow is coming from and try to straw-drink directly from the feeding tube rather than latch onto the breast. It must be cleaned and reassembled frequently. It may be a bit tricky to use away from home. With good support–especially from partners and lactation consultants–these challenges can be overcome and using an at-breast supplementer can become part of your breastfeeding routine.

See the table on previous page to compare advantages and disadvantages of the two most-popular commercially available at-breast supplementers in the United States: Lact-Aid and Supplemental Nursing System (SNS). A homemade at-breast supplementer is much less expensive, but most mothers do not find it convenient for long-term use.

### *How to Use an At-breast Supplementer*

Using an at-breast supplementer is more complicated than the other supplementation devices, though it will likely become routine with some practice. After filling the bag or bottle with human milk or formula and placing it around your neck or beside you, align the feeding tube with the end of your nipple. Some babies do better when the tubing enters their mouth between the philtrum (indent between the nose and upper lip) and the corner of their mouth. Other babies do better when the feeding tube is positioned so that it rests on baby's tongue when they are latched.

Choose a placement of the tubing that is most acceptable to your baby, results in the best latch, and discourages baby from drinking directly from the tubing like a straw (Genna, 2009). The feeding tube

199

can extend to the end of your nipple. Once baby starts suckling, human milk or formula should start immediately moving through the tubing. If the milk or formula doesn't begin to move through the tubing, check that baby is latched well and that the tubing is positioned optimally. Some mothers find it helpful to hold the tubing in place with a finger, surgical tape, or a bandage with adhesive sides trimmed so that the tubing slides under the non-adhesive gauze part. If desired, the bandage may remain on the breast all day so that the tubing can be slipped in and out at each feeding. Using an at-breast supplementer can take some practice for both mother and baby; if it is not working well, use another feeding method for a feeding or two and try again later. If you choose a commercial brand, it will come with additional detailed instructions regarding assembly, use, and cleaning.

If you choose to use an at-breast supplementer, offer the breast without the supplementer at least once or twice a day. If your baby never breastfeeds without the at-breast supplementer, he may refuse the breast without it even when he doesn't need supplementation.

## Bottle

A bottle is the most familiar infant-feeding device in our culture, and it is likely to be the feeding tool your baby is used to if he has not been breastfed from birth. Bottles are socially acceptable in public. They can be easy to find, inexpensive, and easy to clean.

### *How to Bottle-Feed*

Because most of us have seen mothers bottle-feeding since we were children, we may think that we know how to do it. Actually, the way we have seen most mothers bottle-feed may not be in the best interest of your breastfeeding (or soon-to-be-breastfeeding) baby. The bottle-feeding techniques presented in Chapter 8 can help you to use a bottle to transition your baby to breastfeeding, decrease the chance of nipple confusion if your baby is already breastfeeding, and ensure that your baby is not drinking more from the bottle than is necessary.

## Kelly's Story: Supplementing 100%

*Kelly chose to supplement baby Mira with bottles. Because Mira was taking about 32 ounces each day in a bottle, Kelly knew that Mira's time at breast several times throughout the day was for comfort only. Kelly reported that Mira loved to snuggle at the breast, and would tug at Kelly's shirt to let her know she wanted to nurse.*

## Finger-Feeding

With finger-feeding, just as with the at-breast supplementer, the baby receives the supplement through a tiny feeding tube. Instead of the feeding tube at the breast as with the at-breast supplementer, the feeding tube is on the mother's (or other caregiver's) finger. As the baby suckles on the finger, he receives a slow flow of human milk or formula. Because this method of supplementing is rather time-consuming, it is not a preferred long-term method of supplementation. It can be very helpful, though, in transitioning baby to the breast:

- **Finger-feeding can be used to calm baby's hunger before offering the breast.** As discussed in Chapter 7, Finally… Latching!, a baby is more likely to be willing to try the new skill of breastfeeding if he isn't too hungry.
- **Finger-feeding can be used to practice good suckling.** Dr.

Jack Newman (2012) describes how finger-feeding is more like breastfeeding than bottle-feeding.

In order to finger feed, the baby must keep his tongue down and forward over the gums, his mouth wide (the larger the finger used, the better so using a baby finger to do finger feeding is not a good idea), and his jaw forward. Furthermore, the motion of the tongue and jaw is similar to what the baby does while feeding at the breast.

As the baby suckles on your finger, he calms, organizes his suck, and starts to fill his tummy. He is primed for breastfeeding. Once baby has settled into finger-feeding, consider transferring the feeding tube from the finger to the breast, thus shifting the supplementation technique from finger-feeding to at-breast supplementation.

### How to Finger Feed

Finger-feeding devices are available commercially, such as the Hazelbaker FingerFeeder by Aiden and Eva. Alternatively, many lactation consultants will create a homemade finger-feeding device using a 5-French feeding tube. The feeding tube can be placed in a baby bottle and threaded through the bottle nipple if a slightly larger hole is cut out at the tip. If your baby is not able to pull the supplement through the tubing with the end resting in the bottle, connect the feeding tube to a luer-lock syringe; the plunger on the syringe can be pressed to deliver boluses of human milk or formula through the tubing. Alternately, some mothers will use a commercial at-breast supplementer with the feeding tube at the finger rather than the breast; however, the flow from the commercial at-breast supplementer

202

may be very slow since these supplementation devices are designed to augment (some amount of) milk flowing from the breast.

The Hazelbaker FingerFeeder comes with detailed instructions, and your lactation consultant can help with the homemade finger-feeder. The basics are as follows.

Cradle baby in one arm.
- If you are using the Hazelbaker FingerFeeder, the entire device can be held in the hand you are feeding from.
- If you are using a syringe, hold the syringe in the hand of the arm cradling the baby.
- If you are using a bottle, place the bottle on a nearby table, in your shirt breast pocket, or nestled in your bra.

Place the feeding tube along the forefinger of the hand not cradling the baby, nail facing down and the feeding tube placed along the finger almost to the tip. Use your thumb or some surgical tape to hold the tube in place. Tickle the baby's lips with this finger. Wait for the baby to open his mouth wide, allow him to pull the finger into his mouth as far as about your first finger joint. This should be about where the tip of your finger almost reaches the junction of the baby's hard and soft palate. If your baby is able to pull the supplement through the tubing, he will pace the feeding with his suckling rhythm. If he is not able to pull the supplement through the tubing, gently squeeze the bulb of the Hazelbaker FingerFeeder or press the plunger on the syringe when he actively suckles. Stop squeezing/pressing when the baby stops suckling or shows any signs of distress (fingers splaying, wide eyes, furrowed forehead, rapid breathing, or color changes).

Some mothers begin with the feeding tube and syringe and advance to the feeding tube and bottle. Your lactation consultant can provide you with the necessary equipment for finger-feeding and help you get started.

## My Story: Finger-feeding in the Hospital

*By the time Rosa was born, I was pumping about 15 ounces per day, more than enough for her those first few days. Unfortunately, hospital policy required that Rosa was fed her birthmother's milk or infant formula. Since her birthmother had no intention of breastfeeding or expressing her milk during the hospital stay (which in the long run was for the best), Rosa was fed formula in the hospital. I was concerned about nipple confusion (and didn't yet know about the bottle-feeding techniques that support breastfeeding). The lactation consultant at the hospital suggested finger-feeding. She showed me how to do it and it worked just fine for the small amounts of formula Rosa needed for those first two days of life in the hospital. I can't tell you how many questions I received from both*

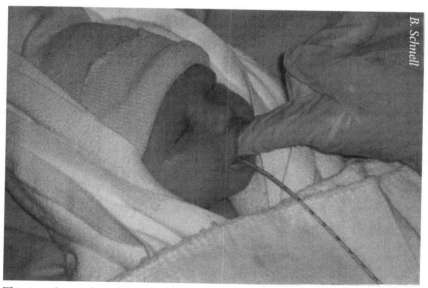

*B. Schnell*

This is a photo of me finger-feeding Rosa during her hospital stay.

*family and hospital staff about why in the world was I feeding the baby this way! Nevertheless, Rosa took immediately to breastfeeding when we got home. We never finger-fed again after that.*

*As I attempted to finger-feed, I noticed that Rosa's tongue did not extend over her lower gum line. As an experienced breastfeeding mother and a La Leche League leader at the time, I knew baby's tongue needs to extend past the gums in order to breastfeed properly. I didn't want to create any bad habits, so I called in the hospital-based lactation consultant. I explained that I wasn't finger-feeding properly because her tongue wasn't extending far enough. The lactation consultant informed me that it wasn't incorrect finger-feeding technique: Rosa was tongue-tied. From across the room, Rosa's birthmother exclaimed, "Oh, I had that, too!" While Rosa was still in the hospital, I was able to make an appointment with a dentist to release her tongue-tie a few days after we returned home —saving us from some potentially major breastfeeding difficulties.*

## Cup Feeding

Even newborn babies can be fed from a cup. Special cups for feeding babies are commercially available, or you can use any small cup, such as a medicine cup or shot glass. Cup-feeding is commonly used for supplementing babies in developing countries, because cups are inexpensive and easy to clean in less-than-ideal conditions.

### How to Cup Feed

Hold baby in a semi-upright position, supporting the shoulders, neck, and head with one hand. A cloth diaper or wash cloth under baby's neck will catch spills. Rest the cup (or a spoon if baby a less than a few days old) filled with human milk or formula on the baby's lower lip. Tip the cup up just enough to bring the milk/formula

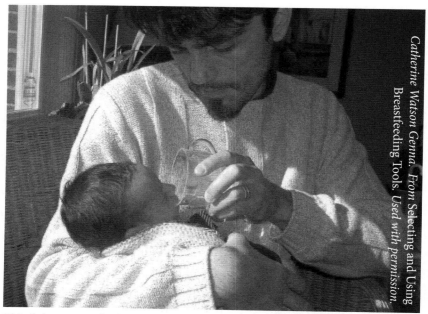

*Catherine Watson Genna. From Selecting and Using Breastfeeding Tools. Used with permission.*

This father is cup-feeding his baby. Note that the baby is fairly upright and the expressed milk or formula is just at the level of baby's lips.

supplement to the edge of the cup. Do not pour the milk or formula into the baby's mouth: allow the baby to lap it like a kitten. The baby may need several breaks when first learning this technique.

Lapping human milk or formula from a cup helps baby practice extending his tongue, a skill necessary for breastfeeding. Cup feeding is unique among the supplementation techniques, because the baby isn't suckling. If a baby is resisting the breast, offering him his supplement via cup means that the only way he can meet his need to suck is to finally breastfeed.

## Pacifier

Even though most people don't typically think of the pacifier as a supplement to breastfeeding, it actually is a substitute for comfort nursing. Babies who use a pacifier spend less time breastfeeding.

More time at the breast, even when baby is not actively suckling for nourishment, means more milk production. It also means more bonding time with your baby.

# Chapter 14

## YOU ARE A BREASTFEEDING MOTHER

No matter how breastfeeding goes for you, whether you latch your baby or not, whether you make no milk or lots of milk, YOU ARE A BREASTFEEDING MOTHER.

## Successful Breastfeeding

### Success is Not Measured by Whether your Baby Ever Latches On

If your baby is never able to latch onto the breast, the tools for latching and attaching, and the process of working towards breastfeeding have brought you and your baby closer to each other. That is what really matters.

> [I]n the process of working towards breastfeeding, mothers have described how they became highly sensitized to their child's emotional well-being. Thus, even mothers whose children never breastfed have stated that they appreciate the sensitivity that working towards breastfeeding developed in them and that they feel that their attempts to facilitate breastfeeding assisted the development of the child-mother relationship (Gribble, 2006, p. 8).

## Success is Not Measured by How Much Milk You Make

Even mothers who enter into breastfeeding without birthing with realistic expectations can feel disappointed when they are not able to make as much milk as they had hoped. If this is your situation, I am here to tell you that you are still a successful breastfeeding mother!

If, despite all the best information and help, you aren't able to make a full milk supply, *you can still breastfeed successfully.* There are many mothers who nurse very satisfactorily with a partial milk supply. They supplement to make up for the amount of milk they can't make, but their main focus is on the milk they can make. They look at the breast as "half full" rather than "half empty"—it's all in how you think about it. One mother with an unusual condition could produce only about a 1 teaspoon (5 ml) of milk each day. She thought of the milk as medicine for her baby, which she proudly gave him each day.

> Every single drop of your milk that your baby gets is wonderfully beneficial, containing all the immunities of a full milk supply and many, many elements completely absent from formula (Wiessinger et al., 2010, p. 16).

# How You Can Help Other Mothers and Babies

Your breastfeeding-without-birthing experience can go a long way toward helping other mother and baby pairs. Spread the word that breastfeeding is possible even for mothers who have not been pregnant. Many adoptive, intended, foster, and non-gestational lesbian mothers don't breastfeed because they never knew it was possible.

Many mothers by birth who wish they were breastfeeding, but are not, may not know it's not too late. Their doctors may not know either.

You can also help others by letting them know that breastfeeding isn't all or nothing, that it is not necessary to exclusively nurse your baby from the breast to be a breastfeeding mother. Breastfeeding-without-birthing mothers are not alone in their breastfeeding struggles, especially with regard to making enough milk. Your breastfeeding experiences can help other mothers in your situation, as well as other mothers with other types of breastfeeding challenges.

Here we are at the end, which I hope for you and your baby is really just the beginning of a wonderful mothering and breastfeeding journey. Best of luck.

*"Mom, you sure are lucky you got an adopted kid."*
-Rosa, now age 7.

# Appendix A

# TIPS FOR PUMPING SUCCESS

Using a breast pump is a learned skill. Unlike breastfeeding, it is not natural or instinctual. Responding to your precious baby suckling at your breast, the feel of his downy hair, that new baby smell, his gurgles and coos, and his hands kneading your breasts trigger your milk to flow. Understandably, you may not respond as well to a cold, hard machine. Fortunately, breastfeeding mothers and their support people have discovered numerous tricks for getting the most from pumping. No mother finds all (or even most) of these tips helpful, but I hope that you will find a few that make your pumping experience as successful and positive as possible.

## Basic Tips

### Tip 1: Rent your pump from a reliable source.

Multi-user breast pumps are available for purchase or rental, although due to their expense most mothers choose to rent[1]. These

[1] Insurance companies are providing better coverage than ever before for the purchase and rental of breast pumps. Check with your insurance carrier whether they will reimburse for the purchase or rental of a multi-user breast pump. If so, you may need a prescription from your doctor. You may also need to obtain the breast pump from a durable medical equipment (DME) provider rather than from the sources listed above. Your insurance carrier will provide a list of DMEs. Even if the purchase or rental of a breast pump is not reimbursed by your insurance carrier, your costs are tax deductible.

pumps may be available through a variety of sources: lactation consultants in private practice, hospital pharmacies, baby boutiques, and drug stores. Your local lactation consultant in private practice, hospital, or La Leche League leader can help direct you to the resources in your area. Once you've got a list of breast-pump rental stations in your area, here are questions you may want to ask before renting.

- **Which breast pumps do you rent?** In general, multi-user breast pumps are quality pumps, but it may be helpful to educate yourself about which are available in your area.
- **What rental terms are available?** The rental terms may be monthly, weekly, or daily.
- **What is the rental fee?**
- **What is the cost of a personal kit?** Multi-user refers to the motor of the breast pump only; you will still need to purchase your own personal kit to use with the pump.
- **How do you test your pumps between renters to ensure they are working properly?** Between each renter, the rental station should test each breast pump with a suction gage to ensure that the pump is reaching a suction level of at least -200 mm/Hg, and that the motor is running smoothly and consistently at various settings.
- **How do you clean your pumps between renters?** I have heard stories of mothers renting a pump that came with another mother's milk splashed all over it – yuck! The pump rental station should wipe down each pump with a disinfectant wipe or cleanser between users.
- **Will you show me how to use the pump?** You should have access to an instructional manual for your pump, either with your pump or online. Even so, it can be very helpful to have

someone experienced with the breast pump show you how to use it the first time. Many of the mothers I work with who are inducing lactation will pick up a breast pump from me on the day they are ready to begin pumping so that the first time they pump, I am there to help.

- **Do you carry various sizes and styles of flanges, and can you help fit me with the appropriate flanges?** (See next tip for more information.)
- **What happens if I have any problems with or questions about the pump?** If you are having difficulties with your pump, the rental station should offer you prompt and reliable assistance.

## Tip 2:  Use properly fitting flanges.

Flanges, also called breast shields or cups, are the part of the breast pump kit that comes in contact with your breasts. Although your breast pump kit comes with one (or possibly two) flange sizes, several sizes and styles of flanges are available for your multi-user breast pump. (The exception is PJ's Comfort breast pump by Limerick. This breast pump uses a flexible silicone flange made to accommodate all mothers.) Using a properly fitting flange will maximize your output and comfort from the pump (Kassing, 2010). Many lactation consultants are trained to fit you with flanges.

## Tip 3:  Optimize breast-pump settings.

Even for mothers who have breastfed or pumped for previous babies, inducing lactation with a breast pump can be rough on nipples. Start slowly and gently with short pumping sessions: only about five minutes or so. It may also help to use a lower suction level at first. If your breast pump has a separate cycle speed setting, you may find it more comfortable at first to set the cycle speed on your breast pump for faster cycles so that the suction on your nipple is held for just a short time each cycle. Over time, your nipples will be acclimated to the stimulation of the breast pump and you will be able to increase your pumping time to 15 to 20 minutes, raise the suction level, and increase the length of the cycles if that makes the pump more effective for you.

The lack of milk flow can also cause discomfort at first. Some mothers choose to hand express for a couple of weeks in order to initiate milk production and then switch to the breast pump. In addition to being an effective way to jump start milk production, hand expressing for a couple of weeks before pumping is a gentler way to introduce regular nipple stimulation.

Once your nipples are acclimated to the breast pump, find the settings that offer you the most comfort and the most output in the shortest amount of time. Because different mothers respond to different stimuli, the pump settings can be different from mother to mother. If the highest comfortable suction level is quite a bit less than the maximum suction level on your pump, this may be an indication that your flanges do not fit properly. Finding the optimal settings for you is a little trickier than it sounds because at first there will be little to no milk. Over time, the amount of milk you produce will increase, and you can make adjustments to the breast-pump settings if necessary.

**Tip 4: Use lubrication as needed.**

If you have the properly-fitted flanges and have found your best settings on the pump and still feel some discomfort, use lubrication. Apply 100% extra virgin olive oil or a commercial nipple cream as a lubricant as needed. Lansinoh brand lanolin is not recommended for this purpose because it is tacky rather than slippery.

**Tip 5: Express your milk frequently.**

For mothers who are exclusively pumping (as in Step 2 of inducing lactation), the key is to simulate the nursing patterns of a baby who is establishing his mother's milk production. A newborn baby nurses at least 8 to 10 times per day, so it is essential to pump this frequently: at least eight times per day on a regular basis. It is important that one of the pumping sessions happens during the middle of the night. Although it is ideal to completely empty the breast each time you pump, pumping for 5 to 10 minutes is more beneficial than not pumping at all.

Some situations in which you might pump even more often are a Pumping Holiday and Power Pumping, which last for no more than a few days at a time. These are both excellent strategies for using pumping frequency to give your milk production a boost. (See Chapter 11, Physical Techniques for Inducing Lactation, for details.)

**Tip 6: Pump with one or both hands free.**

Because you may be pumping very frequently, it can be convenient to have one or both of your hands free while you are pumping. When you first start to pump, you may need to hold the flanges to each breast with one hand each. When you become more comfortable, you may be able to free up one hand by holding the flange on the right breast with your left hand while the left flange is held on with left forearm, leaving your right hand free (or vice-versa if you are left-handed). It is also possible to pump completely hands-free using a hands-free bustier or attachment. See my website for list of hands-free pumping products.

### Tip 7: Keep cleaning of pump collection kit and milk storage simple.

For mothers who are pumping many times throughout the day, cleaning the pump collection kit and storing pumped milk after each pumping session is unnecessary. For mothers who are pumping very frequently, or are power pumping, the kit and bottles can sit at a typical room temperature for up to four to six hours. Aim for four hours in warmer temperatures. While the pump kit sits out, cover the kit and bottles with a clean cloth diaper, receiving blanket, or towel. Then, after four to six hours, the milk can be stored in the refrigerator, the pump collection kit parts are washed, and you are ready to go for the next four to six hours (Genna, 2009).

Another approach is to detach the pump collection kit and attached bottles from the tubing. Place the pair of kits/bottles in a zippered plastic storage bag in the refrigerator between pumping sessions for up to 12 hours at a time before cleaning pump collection kit and storing the expressed milk. Before pumping with refrigerated kit, detach flanges and run under warm water before pumping; applying chilled flanges to the breast can decrease the effectiveness and efficiency of the breast pump (Kent et al., 2011).

Some mothers find having a second pump-collection kit is worthwhile. One kit is air-drying while the second is in use.

# Additional Tips

For many mothers, the basic pumping techniques above will give the results you are looking for. If you are one of those lucky mothers, feel free to skip right over this section. However, if you are finding pumping challenging or you are not getting the output you are looking for, listed below are some additional tips.

## Tip 8: Use Hands-On pumping.

Hands-On pumping simply refers to using breast massage during pumping and/or hand expression after pumping. If you are not getting the output you'd like from your pump, Hands-On pumping is a very effective method for increasing the amount of milk you express. In one study of mothers of preterm babies, 86% of the mothers found that breast massage during pumping, and hand expression after pumping, increased the amount of milk they were able to express by 93% (Morton et al., 2009). Another study found breast massage (without hand expression) during pumping increased the amount of milk they expressed by 42% (Jones et al., 2001). Hands-On pumping is described in detail in Chapter 11, Physical Techniques for Inducing Lactation. Also, see my Links page for a video demonstration of Hands-On pumping.

## Tip 9: Distract yourself.

While pumping, do not watch the bottles. Sometimes it helps to throw a receiving blanket over the kit and bottles. An enjoyable activity while pumping (watching a movie, reading, talking on the phone, listening to music or nature sounds) can distract you and take off some of the pressure.

**Tip 10: Increase relaxation.**

Increase relaxation while pumping. You know what helps you relax: deep breaths, an enjoyable activity, or a scented candle. There are even hypnosis CDs or MP3 downloads to help with relaxation, milk production, and pumping output. (See the Products, page on my website for ordering information.)

**Tip 11: Use visualization.**

It can help to visualize your milk flowing, or a waterfall flowing freely, or whatever image helps you.

**Tip 12: Use sensory inputs.**

When the baby nurses, mother receives many sensory inputs from the baby that help trigger her milk to flow. For many mothers, using sensory stimuli that remind her of her baby can help while pumping: a picture of her baby, a recording of her baby's sounds, or the scent of an unwashed baby blanket or piece of clothing. If your baby hasn't arrived yet, consider sensory inputs that make you think of your baby-to-be. You could pump in your nursery, if you have one. You may have a picture of your baby–even if it's an ultrasound. You could listen to lullabies. Whatever connects you with your baby-to-be.

**Tip 13: Boost your oxytocin.**

Oxytocin is the hormone that causes the milk to eject, also known as let-down. Letting down for a breast pump can be much more difficult than letting down for your baby. In addition to sensory inputs, try things that boost your oxytocin. Having your partner massage you while you are pumping–between the shoulder blades works especially well–will release oxytocin. Laughter and feelings of romance boost oxytocin. Consider reading books or watching movies while you pump that are funny or romantic. One mother found that simply pumping with her husband in the room increased her milk output!

### Tip 14: Apply a warm compress to your breasts before pumping.

A warm compress, such as a warm, moist washcloth can help the milk to flow. Or, make a warm compress by filling a tube sock with rice, knotting the open end, and warming in the microwave. Apply to the breasts just before pumping.

### My Story: Pumping to Induce Lactation

*For the six weeks before Rosa was due, I pumped eight times per day, each day producing more milk than the one before. By the time she arrived, I was pumping 15 ounces per day! I believe that my pumping success was due to a combination of factors. First, I rented a breast pump from a local IBCLC in private practice. She showed me how to use the pump and she fit me with the proper flanges. Then, because I knew that we would have a long and intimate relationship, I named my breast pump. (Lucy, if you must know!) I set up my pumping station in the future nursery. It was comfortable and cozy, with a place for a glass of water and a book. Everything about that room connected me with my baby-to-be. My intention was that being in the nursery would also offer privacy. However, by the second day of pumping, my 3rd grader came in to ask for help with his homework. Pumping isn't very discreet, so I was uncomfortable about an older child witnessing it. But he wasn't uncomfortable, and in the end I think that it helped that I could make pumping flexible around the other needs of the family.*

*In addition to all of the ways the nursery connected my senses with my baby, I was surprised to find how strongly I responded to the smell of my own milk. That smell was what I associated with baby smell.*

*At each pumping session, I double pumped for about 15 minutes. Then I stopped pumping to "massage, stroke, shake" to elicit another letdown. I pumped again for another five minutes or so.*

*I wanted pumping to be as relaxing and enjoyable as possible, and for me that meant fun books to read while pumping. Reading also distracted me from watching the bottles. Prior to inducing lactation, I was always a mystery reader. Yet, while I was pumping, I preferred funny romantic novels. Hmm ... laughter and feelings of romance boost oxytocin, the hormone responsible for milk release.*

*I didn't use all of the techniques suggested in the chapter, but I found just the right ones for me.*

# Appendix B

# DOMPERIDONE: "THE IDEAL GALACTOGOGUE"

Of all of the galactogogues presented in Chapter 12, Medications for Inducing Lactation, Domperidone is by far the most effective in increasing milk production. It is also the safest pharmaceutical galactogogue currently available. Its effectiveness and safety have earned it the designation "ideal galactogogue" by Dr. Thomas Hale, considered to be the world's expert on the use of medications for the breastfeeding mother (Hale, 2012, p. 359). Unfortunately, controversy around this medication has raised concerns both about its safety and its legality. I hope to put some of these concerns to rest for you.

## Domperidone is Safe for Breastfeeding Mothers

Old reports of very ill, elderly patients taking Domperidone intravenously in large doses for gastrointestinal difficulties indicate that the use of Domperidone can have very serious heart-related side effects. Domperidone has not been available in the intravenous form for about 20 years and, when taken orally, Domperidone has never been reported to cause heart-related issues (Wight, 2011). In fact, Domperidone has been widely used by breastfeeding mothers in Canada since the mid-1980s, and Health Canada has never received an adverse action report regarding serious heart-related difficulties "in relation to the use of Domperidone used to stimulate milk production in breastfeeding women" (CBC News, 2012). Domperidone is approved for use in over 80 countries including the Canada, Mexico, the European Union, Australia, and New Zealand. It is available over-the-counter without a prescription in many countries including Belgium, Ireland, Italy, Netherlands, United Kingdom, Switzerland, China, South Africa, Mexico, New Zealand, Chile, and Pakistan (West & Marasco, 2009; Wight, 2011).

Clinical trials are underway (at the time of this writing) to further examine the safety of Domperidone for breastfeeding mothers. Until more information is available, Domperidone is not recommended for mothers:

> ... with a history of known or suspected cardiac arrhythmias (tachyarrhythmia, QT prolongation); currently on an anti-arrhythmic medication; or having a chronic/debilitating illness, abnormal liver function, or serious gastric abnormality. Caution should also be used in mothers concomitantly taking medications known to alter the metabolism of Domperidone (via inhibiting the cytochrome P450 pathway), medications that have dopaminergic or antidopaminergic activity, and medications that may increase the QT interval5 (Flanders et al., 2012).

Mothers who experience heart palpitations, dizziness, fainting, or seizures should stop taking the medication and get medical help immediately (Flanders, 2012).

As with all pharmaceutical medications, Domperidone does have some side effects. They are not serious and usually temporary (Flanders et al., 2012). Side effects in breastfeeding mothers can include dry mouth, transient skin rash or itching, headache, thirst, abdominal cramps, diarrhea, drowsiness, and nervousness. Some mothers find the side effects resolve more quickly when they decrease the dosage, and then gently increase it over time. Other mothers find these effects are minimized when the Domperidone is taken with food.

## Domperidone is Safe for Breastfeeding Babies

The American Academy of Pediatrics (AAP; 2001) lists Domperidone as a medication compatible with breastfeeding. Domperidone has a lactation risk rating of L1, which places it in the category of safest medications for the breastfeeding infant. No known adverse effects on babies have been reported in babies whose mothers have taken Domperidone (Hale, 2012). It is a medication that has been given to infants with reflux in Canada since the mid-1980s, and the amount the baby receives through milk is very small compared to the prescribed dosage for babies with reflux.

## The Process for FDA Approval of Domperidone is Underway

Due to the tireless efforts of the lactation community, Domperidone has been granted orphan drug status and is now in clinical trials, its next step toward FDA approval. Because it is not yet FDA approved, Domperidone is currently not available through most pharmacies. In the meantime, mothers are obtaining Domperidone from certain compounding pharmacies or ordering it from an overseas pharmaceutical distributer. Ordering Domperidone through compounding pharmacies can be much more expensive, and the medication may not always be prepared correctly. Some indications that your medication was not properly compounded are the lack of desired breast changes or developing an itchy rash (L. Goldfarb, personal communication, September 24, 2012). When ordered overseas, your medication can take a couple of weeks to arrive. Talk with your local lactation consultant to see if there is a local pharmacy that will compound Domperidone, or refer to the Products, page of my website for information on ordering it overseas.

## Metoclopramide (Reglan) is Not Recommended for Mothers Inducing Lactation

Metoclopramide (trade name Reglan) is a medication that works similarly to Domperidone, to help the body release prolactin, and results in a significant increase in milk production. Unlike Domperidone, Reglan is FDA approved, so a doctor can write a prescription that can be filled in a regular pharmacy. So why not use metoclopramide instead of Domperidone? Metoclopramide penetrates the blood-brain barrier and Domperidone does not. This means that metoclopramide can have serious side effects on the central nervous system, such as depression and dystonia (involuntary body movements). Because these side effects increase with the length of use, metoclopramide is not recommended for long-term use (longer than two or three weeks), as is generally required for mothers inducing lactation. Metoclopramide also crosses into the milk at a higher percentage than Domperidone (Gabay, 2002).

# Appendix C

# POTENTIAL SIDE EFFECTS AND SAFETY CAUTIONS FOR HERBAL GALACTOGOGUES

In general, herbs are safe and health-promoting methods of supporting lactation. However, herbs are still a type of medication and should be used with some caution. As with any medication, discontinue use if you observe negative side effects.

The Humphrey Safety Ratings have been designated by herbalist, nurse, and lactation consultant Sheila Humphrey (Humphrey, 2003, p. 272). The Humphrey Safety Ratings are as follows:

A. No contraindications, side effects, drug interactions, or pregnancy-related safety issues have been identified. Generally considered safe when used appropriately.

B. May not be appropriate for self-use by some individuals or dyads, or may cause adverse effects if misused. Seek reliable safety and dose information.

C. Moderate potential for toxicity, mainly dose related. Seek an expert herbalist as well as a lactation consultation before using. Consider using safer herbs.

| Herb | Humphrey Safety Rating | Potential Side Effects and Safety Concerns |
|---|---|---|
| Alfalfa (plant) | A | May cause diarrhea. If so, temporarily reduce dosage. |
| Alfalfa (seed) | C | Persons with lupus or other autoimmune disorder should avoid. |
| Blessed Thistle | B | Potential allergen (rare).<br><br>Appetite stimulant.<br><br>Stimulates gastric juices. Persons with ulcers, hyperacidity, or acute stomach inflammation should use with caution. |
| Fennel | A | Potential allergen (very rare).<br>May suppress appetite. |
| Fenugreek | B | Appetite stimulant.<br>Urine and sweat may smell like maple syrup.<br>May trigger asthma or wheezing.<br><br>Occasional side effects are nausea, faintness, diarrhea, or running sinuses that usually discontinue after a few days. It may help to decrease dosage and gradually build.<br><br>Other potential side effects are migraine headaches, high blood pressure, decreased blood sugar, and decreased thyroid level.<br><br>Use under the guidance of your doctor if you are on blood-thinning medication, or have hypoglycemia, diabetes, or hypothyroidism. |
| Goat's Rue | B | Helps to balance blood sugar and may increase sensitivity to insulin. Use under the guidance of your doctor if you have diabetes or hypoglycemia. |
| Saw Palmetto | A | |
| Shatavari | B | |

Information in the above table was taken from *The Nursing Mother's Herbal* (Humphrey), *Motherfood* (Jacobson), and *The Breast-feeding Mother's Guide to Making More Milk* (West & Marasco). For more information on these herbs, please refer to any of these excellent resources.

# REFERENCES

AAP Committe on Drugs. (2001). The transfer of drugs and other chemicals into human milk. *Pediatrics, 108*(3), 776-789.

Abejide, O.R., Tadese, M.A., Babajide, D.E., Torimiro, S.E., Davies-Adetugbo, A.A., & Makanjuola, R.O. (1997). Non-puerperal induced lactation in a Nigerian community: Case reports. *Annals of Tropical Paediatrics, 17*(2), 109-114.

American Academy of Pediatrics. (2005). Breastfeeding and the use of human milk. *Pediatrics, 115*(2), 496-506.

American Congress of Obstetricians and Gynecologists. (2007). Breastfeeding: Maternal and infant aspects. *ACOG Committee Opinion No. 361, 109*, 479-480.

Amico, J. A., & Finley, B. E. (1986). Breast stimulation in cycling women, pregnant woman and a woman with induced lactation: Pattern of release of oxytocin, prolactin, and luteinizing hormone. *Clinical Endocrinology, 25*(2), 97-106. doi:10.1111/j.1365-2265.1986.tb01670.x

Auerbach, K., & Avery, J. L. (1981). Induced lactation: A study of adoptive nursing by 240 women. *American Journal of Diseases of Children, 135*, 340-343.

Avery, J. L. (2012). *Frequently asked questions about nursing adopted babies*. Retrieved from: http://www.lact-aid.com/faq-about-nursing-adoptive-babies/

Behrmann, B. L. (2005). *The breastfeeding cafe*. Ann Arbor: The University of Michigan Press.

Berggren, K. (2009). *Just like riding a bike*. Retrieved from: http://www.workandpump.com/bike.htm

Biervliet, F.P., Maguiness, S.D., Hay, D.M., Killick, S.R., & Atkin, S.L. (2001). Induction of lactation in the intended mother of a surrogate pregnancy. *Human Reproduction, 16*(3), 581-583.

Bonyata, K. (2012). *Financial costs of not breastfeeding.* Retrieved from: kellymom.com/pregnancy/bf-prep/bfcostbenefits/

Cassar-Uhl, D. (2012). "Yes, you can breastfeed!" Supporting mothers with mammary hypoplasia/insufficient glandular tissue as a lactation consultant in private practice. *Lactation Consultant in Private Practice Workshop.* Philadelphia.

Caughman, S., & Motley, I. (2009). *You can adopt: An adoptive families guide.* New York: Ballantine Books.

CBC News. (2012). *Domperidone safety alert issued by Health Canada.* Retrieved from: http://www.cbc.ca/news/health/story/2012/03/08/domperidone-maleate-drug-.html

Centers for Disease Control and Prevention. (2009). *Breastfeeding: Diseases and conditions.* Retrieved from: http://www.cdc.gov/breastfeeding/disease/

Cheales-Siebenaler, N. J. (1999). Induced lactation in an adoptive mother. *Journal of Human Lactation, 15*(1), 41-43.

Clark, R.A., Richard-Davis, G., Hayes, J., Murphy, M., & Theall, K.P. (2009). *Planning parenthood: Strategies for success in fertility assistance, adoption, and surrogacy.* Baltimore, MD: The Johns Hopkins University Press.

Cohen, R.S., Xiong, S.C., & Sakamoto, P. (2009). Retrospective review of serological testing of potential human milk donors. *Archives of Diseases of Childhood, Fetal & Neonatal Edition, 95,* F118-F120.

Collaborative Group on Hormonal Factors in Breast Cancer. (2002). Breast cancer and breastfeeding: Collaborative reanalysis of individual data from 47 epidemiological studies in 30 countries, including 50,302 women with breast cancer and 96,973 women without the disease. *Lancet, 350,* 187-195.

Colson, S. (2010). *An introduction to biological nurturing: New angles on breastfeeding.* Amarillo, TX: Hale publishing.

Colson, S. (2012). *Sample of biological nurturing.* Retrieved from: http://www.biologicalnurturing.com/video/bn3clip.html

Cornais, S. (2010). *Make your boobs a happy place.* Retrieved from: http://mamaandbabylove.com/2010/12/31/make-your-boobs-a-happy-place/

Creating a Family. (2012). *Breastfeeding and adoption & surrogacy.* Retrieved from: http://www.creatingafamily.org/adoption/resources.html

Davenport, D. (2009). *Breastfeeding the adopted child.* Retrieved from: http://www.creatingafamily.org/adoption-resources/breastfeeding-the-adopted-child.html#Americanacademy

Davenport, D. (2011). *Breastfeeding the international adopted baby.* Retrieved from: http://www.youtube.com/watch?v=Q-rtnGMl7w0

Dettwyler, K. A. (2003). A time to wean: The hominid blueprint for a natural age of weaning in modern human populations. In P. Stuart-Macadam, & K. A. Dettwyler (Eds.), *Breastfeeding: Biocultural perspectives* (pp. 39-73). New York: Aldine De Gruyter.

Drummund, P. D., & Hewson-Bower, B. (1997). Increased psycho-social stress and decreased mucosal immunity in children with recurrent upper respiratory tract infections. *Journal of Psychosomatic Research, 43(3),* 271-278.

Field, T.M., Schanberg, S.M., Scafidi, F., Bauer, C.R., Vega-Lahr, N., Garcia, R., Nystrom, J., & Kuhn, C.M. (1986). Tactile/

kinesthetic stimulation effects on preterm neonates. *Pediatrics, 77*(5), 654-658.

Flanders, D., Lowe, A., Kramer, M., da Silva, O., Dobrich, C., Campbell-Yeo, M., Kernerman, E., & Newman, J. (2012). *A consensus statement on the use of domperidone to support lactation.* Retrieved from: http://kindercarepediatrics.ca/wp-content/uploads/Domperidone-Consensus-Statement-Final-May-11-2012.pdf

Flanders, D. (2012). *The (not so) great Canadian domperidone debacle.* Retrieved from: http://kindercarepediatrics.ca/2012/03/the-not-so-great-canadian-domperidone-debacle-%E2%80%93-next-steps/

Gabay, M. P. (2002). Galactogogues: Medications that induce lactation. *Journal of Human Lactation, 18,* 274-279.

Genna, C. W. (2008). *Supporting sucking skills in breastfeeding infants.* Sudbury, MA: Jones and Bartlett.

Genna, C. W. (2009). *Selecting and using breastfeeding tools: Improving care and outcomes.* Amarillo, TX: Hale Publishing.

Genna, C. W. (2011). Non-latching infant first 48 hours and beyond. *Central Illinois Breastfeeding Task Force 2011 Fall Conference.* East Peoria, IL.

Goldfarb, L. (2011). *Breastfeeding the child through adoption or surrogacy.* (D. Davenport, Interviewer) Retrieved from: http://www.creatingafamily.org/radioplayer.html?file_name=breastfeeding%20the%20child.mp3&year=2011%20&day=Feb.%209&title=Breastfeeding%20the%20Child%20Through%20Adoption%20or%20Surrogacy

Granju, K. A., & Kennedy, B. (1999). *Attachment parenting: Instinctive care for your baby and young child.* New York: Pocket Books.

Gribble, K. (2004). Adoptive breastfeeding beyond infancy. *Leaven,*

*40*(5), 99-102.

Gribble, K. (2004). The influence of context on the success of adoptive breastfeeding: Developing countries and the west. *Breastfeeding Review, 12*(1), 5-13.

Gribble, K. (2005). Breastfeeding of a medically fragile foster child. *Journal of Human Lactation, 21*(1), 42-46.

Gribble, K. (2005). Post-institutionalized adopted children who seek breastfeeding from their new mothers. *Journal of Prenatal and Perinatal Psychology and Health, 9*(3), 217-235.

Gribble, K. (2006). Mental health, attachment, and breastfeeding: Implications for adopted children and their mothers. *International Breastfeeding Journal, 1*(5). doi:10.1186/1746-4358-1-5

Gribble, K. D., & Hausman, B. L. (2012). Milk sharing and formula feeding: Infant feeding risks in comparative perspective? *Australasian Medical Journal, 5*(5), 275-283.

Hale, T. W. (2012). *Medications and mothers' milk, 15th edition.* Amarillo, TX: Hale Publishing.

Halfon, N., Mendonca, A., & Berkowitz, G. (1995). Health status of children in foster care: The experience of the Center for the Vulnerable Child. *Archives of Pediatric & Adolescent Medicine, 149*(4), 386-392.

Hormann, E. (1977). Breastfeeding the adopted baby. *Birth and the Family Journal, 4,* 165.

Humphrey, S. (2003). *The nursing mother's herbal.* Minneapolis: Fairview Press.

Ip, S., Chung, M., Raman, G., Chew, P., Magula, N., DeVine, D., Trikalinos, T., & Lau, J. (2007). *Breastfeeding and maternal and infant health outcomes in developed countries: Evidence report/technology assessment no. 157.* Rockville, MD: Agency for Healthcare Research and Quality.

Israel-Ballard, K., Coutsoudis, A., Chantry, C.J., Sturm, A.W., Karim, F., Sibeko, L., & Abrams, B. (2006). Bacterial safety of flash-heated and unheated expressed breastmilk during storage. *Journal of Tropical Pediatrics, 52*(6), 399-405.

Jacobson, H. (2007). *Motherfood: Food and herbs that promote milk production and a mother's health.* Self-published: Rosalind Press.

Jelliffe, D.B., & Jelliffe, E. P. (1972). Non-puerperal induced lactation. *Pediatrics, 50*(1), 170-171.

Jones, E., Dimmock, P.W., & Spencer, S.A. (2001). A randomized controlled trial to compare methods of milk expression after preterm delivery. *Archives of Disease in Childhood. Fetal and Neonatal Edition, 85*(2), F91-F95.

Kam, K. (2008). *No more periods.* Retrieved from: http://www.webmd.com/sex/birth-control/features/no-more-periods

Kassing, D. (2002). Bottle-feeding as a tool to reinforce breastfeeding. *Journal of Human Lactation, 18*(1), 56-60.

Kassing, D. (2010). *Fitting mothers for pump flanges.* La Leche League of Missouri Conference. Columbia, MO.

Kent, J.C., Geddes, D.T., Hepworth, A.R., & Hartmann, P.E. (2011). Effect of warm breastshields on breast milk pumping. *Journal of Human Lactation, 27*(4), 331-338.

Koning, L. (2011). *How two lesbian mamas share breastfeeding duties.* Retrieved from: http://offbeatmama.com/2011/02/co-breast-feeding

Kuhn, K. (1999). *Choosing a breastfeeding-friendly pediatrician.* Retrieved from: http://www.ivillage.com/choosing-breastfeeding-friendly-pediatrician/6-n-145586

Kulski, J. K., Hartmann, P.E., Saint, W.J., Giles, P.F., & Gutteridge,

D.H. (1981). Changes in milk composition of nonpueral women. *American Journal of Obstetrics & Gynecology, 59*(1), 597-604.

Labbok, M. (2000). What is the definition of breastfeeding. *Breastfeeding Abstracts, 19*(3), 19-21.

La Leche League International. (2006). *La Leche League purpose and philosophy.* Retrieved from: La Leche League International: http://www.llli.org/philosophy.html?m=1,0,1

Lee, N. (2011). *Complementary and alternative medicine in breastfeeding therapy.* Amarillo, TX: Hale Publishing.

Marasco, L. (2012). Galactogogues and nutrition: Role of lactogenic food and herbs in milk production. *Breastfeeding: Dealing with the monkey wrenches.* Edwardsville, IL: Edwardsville Region Breastfeeding Task Force Conference.

Marmet, C. (2001). The Marmet Technique of Hand Expression. In D. West, *Defining your own success: Breastfeeding after breast reduction surgery* (pp. 317-320). Schaumburg, IL: La Leche League International.

Maunder, R. G., & Hunter, J. J. (2001). Attachment and psychosomoatic medicine: Development contributions to stress and disease. *Psychosomatic Medicine, 63*(4), 556-567.

May, J. T. (1999). Breastmilk and infection: A brief overview. *Breastfeeding Review, 7*(3), 25-27.

McKenna, J. (2012). *Safe co-sleeping guidelines.* Retrieved from: http://cosleeping.nd.edu/safe-co-sleeping-guidelines/

Meier, P.P., Brown, L.P., Hurst, N.M., Spatz, D.L., Engstrom, J.L., Borucki, L.C., & Krouse, A.M. (2000). Nipple shields for preterm infants: Effect on milk transfer and duration of breastfeeding. *Journal of Human Lactation, 16*(2), 106-114.

Melina, L. R. (1998). *Raising adopted children: Practical, reassuring advice for every adoptive parent*. New York, NY: HarperCollins Publishers, Inc.

Moberg, K. U. (2003). *The oxytocin factor: Tapping the hormone of calm, love, and healing*. London: Printer and Martin Ltd.

Mohrbacher, N. (2010). *Breastfeeding answers made simple*. Amarillo, TX: Hale Publishing.

Mohrbacher, N., & Kendall-Tackett, K. (2005). *Breastfeeding made simple: Seven natural laws for nursing mothers*. Oakland, CA: New Harbinger.

Mohrbacher, N., & Kendall-Tackett, K. (2010). *Breastfeeding made simple: Seven natural laws for breastfeeding mothers, 2nd Ed.* Oakland: New Harbinger Publications, Inc.

Moran, L., & Gilad, J. (2007). From folklore to scientific evidence: Breast-feeding and wet-nursing in Islam and the case of non-pueral lactation. *International Journal of Biomedical Science, 3*(4), 251-257.

Morton, J. (2010). *Hand expression of breastmilk*. Retrieved from: http://newborns.stanford.edu/Breastfeeding/HandExpression.html

Morton, J. (2012). *Maximizing milk production with hands on pumping*. Retrieved from: http://newborns.stanford.edu/Breastfeeding/MaxProduction.html

Morton, J., Wong, R.L., Hall, J.Y., Pang, W.W., Lai, C.T., Lui, J., Hartmann, P.E., & Rhine, W.D. (2009). Combining hand techniques with electric pumping increases milk production in mothers of preterm infants. *Journal of Perinatology, 32*(10), 757-764.

Newman, J. (2011). When the baby has not yet taken the breast. *Central Illinois Breastfeeding Task Force*. East Peoria.

Newman, J. (2009). *Breast compression*. Retrieved from: http://www.

breastfeedinginc.ca/content.php?pagename=doc-BC

Newman, J., & Goldfarb, L. (accessed October 26, 2012). *The proto-cols for induced lactation - a guide for maximising milk production: The regular protocol.* Retrieved from: http://www.asklenore.info/breastfeeding/induced_lactation/regular_protocol.shtml

Newman, J., & Goldfarb, L. (accessed October 31, 2012). *The protocols for induced lactation - a guide for maximising breastmilk production: the menopause protocol.* Retrieved from: http://www.asklenore.info/breastfeeding/induced_lactation/menopause_protocol.shtml

Newman, J., & Goldfarb, L. (accessed July 11, 2012). *Breastfeeding: Special birth control.* Retrieved from: http://www.asklenore.info/breastfeeding/induced_lactation/birth_control.shtml

Newman, J., & Goldfarb, L. (accessed October 26, 2012). *The proto-cols for induced lactation - a guide for maximising milk production: The regular protocol.* Retrieved from: http://www.asklenore.info/breastfeeding/induced_lactation/regular_protocol.shtml

Riordan, J. (2005). *Breastfeeding and human lactation, 3rd edition.* Jones and Bartlett: Boston.

Palmer, B. (2011). *The evolution of malocclusion and sleep apnea.* (S. Y. Park, Interviewer). Retrieved from: http://www.brianpalmerdds.com/

Peterson, A., & Harmer, M. (2010). *Balancing breast & bottle: Reaching your breastfeeding goals.* Amarillo, TX: Hale Publishing.

Pisacane, A., Continisio, G.I., Aldinucci, M., D'Amora, S., & Continisio, P. (2005). A controlled trial of the father's role in breastfeeding promotion. *Pediatrics*, e494-e498.

Powers, D. C., & Tapia, V. B. (2012). Clinical decision making: When to consider a nipple shield. *Clinical Lactation, 3*(1), 26-28.

Schleifer, S.J., Scott, B., Stein, M., & Keller, S.E. (1986). Behavioral and developmental aspects of immunity. *Journal of the American Academy of Child Psychiatry, 25*(6), 751-763.

Schneider, B. (1986). Providing for the health needs of migrant children. *Nurse Practitioner, 2*, 54-58.

Sember, B. M. (2007). *The adoption answer book: Your guide to a successful adoption.* Naperville, IL: Sphinx.

Smillie, C. M. (2008). How infants learn to feed: A neurobehavioral model. In C. W. Genna, *Supporting sucking skills in breastfeeding infants* (pp. 79-95). Boston, MA: Jones and Bartlett.

Starr, D. (2008). *Preparation for adoptive nursing.* Retrieved from: http://www.fourfriends.com/abrw/Darillyn%27s/preparation.htm

Thorley, V. (2004). Breastfeeding culture is important to the success of inducing lactation in the absence of pregnancy or after a gap. *Breastfeeding Review, 12*(3), 27.

Tohotoa, J., Maycock, B., Hauck, Y.L., Howat, P., Burns, S., & Binns, C.W. (2009). Dads make a difference: An exploratory study of paternal support for breastfeeding in Perth, Western Australia. *International Breastfeeding Journal,* 4:15. doi:10.1186/1746-4358-4-15

U.S. Department of Health and Human Services. (accessed January 24, 2013). *Postadoption depression.* Retrieved from Child Welfare Information Gateway: https://www.childwelfare.gov/adoption/adopt_parenting/depression.cfm

U. S. Department of Health and Human Services. (2010). *Consent to adoption.* Retrieved from: https://www.childwelfare.gov/systemwide/laws_policies/statutes/consent.cfm#_note11

U.S. Department of Health and Human Services. (2011). *The Surgeon*

*General's Call to Action to Support Breastfeeding*. Washington, DC: U.S. Department of Health and Human Services, Office of the Surgeon General.

West, D. (2001). *Defining your own success: Breastfeeding after breast reduction surgery*. Schaumburg, IL: La Leche League International.

West, D., & Marasco, L. (2009). *The breastfeeding mother's guide to making more milk*. New York: McGraw Hill.

West, D., & Marasco, L. (2009). *At-breast supplementers*. Retrieved from: http://www.lowmilksupply.org/abs.shtml

West, D., & Marasco, L. (2009). *Is domperidone safe and can it be obtained legally in the U.S.?* Retrieved from: http://www.lowmilk-supply.org/domperidone-safe.shtml

Wiessinger, D. (2008). *Finding a real, live helper*. Retrieved from: Common Sense Breastfeeding: www.normalfed.com

Wiessinger, D., West, D., & Pitman, T. (2010). *The womanly art of breastfeeding, 8th edition*. New York: Ballantine Books.

Wight, N. E. (2011). *Domperidone for improving breastmilk production*. Retrieved from: http://www.breastfeeding.org/uploaded_files/bf_meds/Domperidone_Patient_Handout.pdf

Wilson, M.E., Megel, M.E., Fredrichs, A.M., & McLaughlin, P. (2003). Physiologic and behavioral responses to stress, temperament, and incidence of infection and atopic disorders in the first year of life: A pilot study. *Journal of Pediatric Nursing, 4,* 257-266.

Wolfberg, A.J., Michels, K.B., Shields, W., O'Campo, P., Bronner, Y., & Bienstock, J. (2004). Dads as breastfeeding advocates: Results from a randomized controlled trial of an educational intervention. *American Journal of Obstetrics and Gynecology, 191*(3), 708-712.

World Health Organization. (2003). *Global strategy for infant and young child feeding*. Geneva: World Health Organization.

World Health Organization. (1998). *Relactation: A review of experience and recommendations for practice*. Geneva: The World Health Organization.

World Health Organization, Department of Reproductive Health and Research. (2008). *Progestogen-only contraceptive use during lactation and its effects on the neonate*. Retrieved from World Health Organization: http://www.who.int/reproductivehealth/publications/family_planning/WHO_RHR_09_13/en/index.html

Yang, S. (2007). *HIV in breastmilk killed by flash-heating, new study finds*. Retrieved from: http://www.berkeley.edu/news/media/releases/2007/05/21_breastmilk.shtml

17168207R00135

Printed in Great Britain
by Amazon